ANTI-INFLAMMATORY DIET

Simple Recipes To Heal The Immune System And Reduce Inflammation In 30 Days

KAREN GOMEZ

Table of Contents

Introduction 5

Anti-Inflammatory Diet 6

Most Powerful Anti-Inflammatory Foods 18

    Inflammatory Foods to Avoid 29

30 Day Diet Plan Challenge 30

What Do Vegans Eat? 35

Lists Of Anti-Inflammatory Recipes 43

    1.   Kale smoothie 43

    2.   Grouper in green sauce 45

    3.   Monkfish and spinach parcels 47

    4.   Grilled Hake and Vegetables Recipe 50

    5.   Asparagus and green pea's salad 53

    6.   Rocket salad with mango, avocado and cherry tomatoes 55

    7.   Pumpkin cream 57

    8.   Rocket salad with mango, avocado and cherry tomatoes 59

    3.   Grilled asparagus salad with parmesan 61

    4.   Vegan chakchouka 63

    5.   Vegetable croquettes 65

    6.   Tagine of vegetables with spices 67

    7.   Little Peas, the French Way 69

    8.   Gourmet pea, edamame, and green asparagus salad 71

    9.   Pea salad, gourmet peas, grapefruit 73

    10.   Thai Pumpkin Soup 75

    11.   Dry belly soup with cabbage and celery 77

    12.   Dry Soup Recipe for Pumpkin Belly 79

    13.   Dry belly soup recipe with cabbage 81

    14.   Dry belly soup recipe with sweet potato 83

15.   Pumpkin Soup 85

16.   Cabbage soup 87

Two Sides Of Inflammation 89

The secret cause of inflammation 91

Five horsemen of inflammation 93

The Influence Of Psychosomatic Factors On The Course Of Digestive Diseases 99

Diet In Chronic Kidney Disease 111

Conclusion 124

Introduction

Chronic fatigue, depression, diabetes, obesity, hypertension - chronic inflammation in the body can lead to these problems. How can I stop it? This will help, among other things, an appropriately structured diet.

Inflammation is the body's natural defense response to infection or infection. It is designed to eliminate the source of the threat and correct the "damage." However, if inflammation persists for too long, it in itself becomes a serious threat to our health.

An acute inflammatory process sometimes turns into a chronic one, which can last for months or even years. This leads to constant stimulation of the immune system and tissue destruction in the place where it occurs. The so-called pro-inflammatory cytokines begin to spread through the body's circulatory system, resulting in various ailments, depressed mood, chronic fatigue syndrome, or migraine.

In the long term, the effect of chronic inflammation is even more serious, as it leads to the development of many formidable diseases, in particular, Hashimoto's disease, diabetes mellitus, obesity, vascular atherosclerosis, and even cancer.

The keys success is eliminating foods that support inflammation while adding foods with anti-inflammatory properties.

What anti-inflammatory foods are there? How can they change your health?

Inflammation is a basic function of the body, and it's not always a bad thing. When you are injured or sick, the lymphatic (immune) system kicks in, delivering an army of white blood cells to do affect the area by increasing blood flow. In the diseased area, redness, swelling may occur. You may feel fever, pain, discomfort. You've probably watched a cut or scratch swell and feel hot to the touch as blood rushes to it. In a healthy body, inflammation is a normal and effective response that promotes healing.

But that's not the whole story.

Sometimes the immune system breaks down and then starts attacking healthy tissues in the body. This is a common pattern in autoimmune diseases. Inflammatory effects are also associated with arthritis, fibromyalgia, celiac disease, and IBS (irritable bowel syndrome). In asthma, inflammation of the airways is formed; inflammation in diabetes affects insulin resistance, etc.

Despite the link between inflammation and common diseases, and the link between diet and inflammation, diet is not always recommended as a treatment. The 2014 IBD study is an anti-inflammatory diet, a dietary regimen for inflammatory bowel disease that limits the intake of certain carbohydrates includes prebiotic and probiotic foods, and modifies dietary fatty acids. The diet was offered to 40 patients. 13 of them (33%) chose not to try the diet. 24 (60%) patients had a good or very good response to the diet, and the results of 3 (7%) patients were mixed. 11 patients, aged 19 to 70 years, 8 with Crohn's disease (chronic inflammation, most often affecting the end of the small intestine and then beginning of the colon) and 3 with ulcerative colitis, followed an anti-inflammatory diet for 4 weeks or more. After the diet, all patients were able to stop taking at least one of their medications. All showed a reduction in symptoms.

Anti-inflammatory diet

To move on to an anti-inflammatory diet, you must turn your attention to ancient Mediterranean eating patterns. The Mediterranean diet is high in vegetables and fruits, contains almost no red meat, and is abundant in omega-3 fatty acids. To fight inflammation, fresh foods contain a number of essential nutrients:

- Antioxidants

- Minerals

- Essential fatty acids

The pursuit of a healthy diet begins with a menu high in vegetables, fruits, and sprouted seeds.

Take your time to empty your refrigerator and fly to the Mediterranean to follow ancient, healthy eating habits. You can do this at home by gradually adding healthy foods to the menu and removing unhealthy ones. Gradual changes tend to be more sustainable in the long term and easier to tolerate, which means there is less likelihood of reverting to old eating patterns.

By simply adding foods to your menu that fight inflammation and restore health at the cellular level, you can begin to heal your body without any major changes. Once you find foods that heal the body and satisfy the taste, you can remove all the culprits of inflammation, and you won't feel cheated.

1. Green leafy vegetables

The vegetable drawer is the first thing you should fill in your refrigerator or pantry. Vegetables and fruits are rich in antioxidants that restore cellular health. Add green leafy vegetables to your meals; make salads and juices from them. I can share a recipe for anti-inflammatory juice. For it, you will need:

- 4 stalks of celery
- 1/2 cucumber
- 1 cup pineapple
- 1/2 green apple
- 1 cup spinach
- 1 slice of ginger
- 1 lemon

Pass all the ingredients through a juicer, stir the juice, and drink right away.

The Swiss chard (leaf beet is) a lot of antioxidants, vitamins A, C, and K - that can assist protect your brain from oxidative stress caused by free radicals.

2. Bok Choi

Bok Choi is also known as Pak Choi or Chinese cabbage. It is an excellent source of trace minerals. Research shows that Bok Choi contains over 70 antioxidant phenolic compounds. These include hydroxycinnamic acids, which are powerful free radical scavenging antioxidants.

3. Celery

Recent pharmacological studies have proven the benefits of celery in improving blood pressure, stabilizing cholesterol, and preventing heart disease. Celery seeds have tremendous health benefits, which can be found whole, as an extract, or as a powder. They help reduce inflammation and fight various bacterial infections. It is also a great source of potassium, antioxidants, and vitamins.

The key to a healthy body, like everything else in the world, is balance. A good example of mineral balance associated with inflammation is the right mix of sodium and potassium foods. Sodium provides fluid and nutrients, while potassium removes toxins. We usually eat a lot of foods containing sodium, these are:

- Bakery products
- Pizza
- Sandwiches
- Sausages
- Soups
- Burrito and tacos
- Chips, popcorn, crackers, pretzels
- Chicken
- Cheese

- Egg products

And we practically do not consume foods rich in potassium, and these are:

- Avocado
- Pumpkin Acorn
- Spinach
- Sweet potato
- Wild salmon
- Dried apricots
- Garnet
- Coconut milk
- White beans
- Bananas

Without potassium, toxins will accumulate in the body, fraught with the appearance or increase of already existing inflammation. Celery is an excellent source of potassium.

4. Beets

The characteristic color of beets is given by the antioxidant betalain, which is excellent at fighting inflammation and restoring damaged cells. Beets are rich in potassium and magnesium, and magnesium deficiency is closely associated with inflammatory conditions. Calcium is poorly absorbed without magnesium. Its accumulation in the body is highly undesirable since it can cause calcified kidney stones' appearance and then inflammatory processes. But with a balanced diet rich in calcium and magnesium, the body processes everything and absorbs it.

5. Broccoli

Broccoli is a valuable vegetable in any diet. This cabbage is rich in potassium and magnesium and has powerful antioxidant effects.

The flavonoids, carotenoids, antioxidants, and vitamins found in broccoli work together to reduce oxidative stress in the body, help fight chronic inflammation, and reduce cancer risk.

6. Blueberries

One of the powerful antioxidants is quercetin. It is found in citrus fruits, olive oil, and dark berries. The presence of quercetin and other phytonutrient anthocyanins (the so-called water-soluble vacuolar pigments that give the product its red, purple, or blue color) make blueberries very healthy.

Research shows that eating large amounts of blueberries slows down cognitive decline, improves memory and physical activity.

7. Pineapple

Pineapple contains a digestive enzyme called bromelain. An RCT investigated the immunomodulatory activity of bromelain at low and high doses after oral administration. For the first time, bromelain has been shown to modulate lymphocytes' cellular responses and have a powerful anti-inflammatory effect.

Anance helps improve blood clotting rates and protects the heart as well as aspirin. Bromelain prevents the clumping and buildup of platelets on blood vessels' walls, which is a known cause of heart attacks, including strokes.

Pineapple is high in vitamin C, B1, potassium, manganese, and other antioxidants, phytonutrients that reduce the symptoms of some common diseases.

8. Walnuts

Walnuts are also a source of omega-3s. Add them to a salad drizzled with olive oil for a hearty, tasty anti-inflammatory meal, or grab a handful for a snack. Some phytonutrients found in walnuts are very difficult to find in other foods.

Thanks to them, walnuts can protect against metabolic syndrome, cardiovascular disease, and type 2 diabetes.

9. Coconut oil

Much can be written about how herbs and oils work in tandem to provide anti-inflammatory benefits. Lipids and spices create powerful anti-inflammatory compounds. This is especially true for coconut oil and curcumin. The high levels of antioxidants are present in virgin coconut oil reduced inflammation and treated arthritis more effectively than advanced drugs.

The main culprits of osteoporosis are oxidative stress and free radicals.

Since coconut oil benefits include its ability to fight free radicals, it is becoming the leading natural treatment for osteoporosis.

10. Chia seeds

Chia seeds contain omega-3 including omega-6 fatty acids that should be consumed in a 1: 1 ratio to maintain balance.

Chia is a natural antioxidant with an anti-inflammatory effect, containing essential fatty acids alpha-linolenic and linoleic acids, mucin, strontium, vitamins A, B, E, D, as well as sulfur, iron, iodine, magnesium, manganese, niacin, thiamine. When oxidative stress is reversed, it will decrease the likelihood of developing atherosclerosis, so consuming chia seeds regularly is a good idea.

Add a tablespoon of seeds to a jar of natural yogurt that I make at home. This can be not only a great snack but also a complete meal.

11. Flax seeds

Lignans are unique fiber-linked polyphenols with antioxidant properties for rejuvenation, hormonal balance, and cellular health—an excellent source of omega-3 fatty acids.

Polyphenols assist the growth of probiotics in the intestines and help eliminate pathogenic yeast and candidiasis in the body.

Add them to yogurt; only before that, you need to grind them in a coffee grinder to make it easier for the digestive tract to work.

12. Turmeric

Curcumin has long been known in the East and belongs to anti-inflammatory spices. It is documented that turmeric is incredibly healthy for inflammation and is essential in an anti-inflammatory diet.

Aspirin and ibuprofen were found to be less effective in providing anti-inflammatory and ant proliferative properties than curcumin.

Turmeric helps people cope with rheumatoid arthritis. A recent study from Japan assessed its association with interleukin-6, an inflammatory cytokine involved in rheumatoid arthritis, and found that curcumin significantly reduced a marker of inflammation.

13. Ginger

Ginger is useful in any form - fresh, dry, in supplements and extracts - and is an excellent immunomodulatory. Eastern medicine has appreciated the properties of ginger. She believes that because ginger warms the body effectively, it can help break down accumulated toxins. Also, it cleanses the lymphatic system. Ginger can safely take part in the treatment of inflammation in allergic and asthmatic disorders.

Inflammatory foods

The main food you should eliminate is Trans fats. Found in processed foods, they cause inflammation, obesity, diabetes, and cardiovascular disease.

It is also necessary to exclude foods that contain more omega-6 than necessary. In excess and out of balance with omega-3s, omega-6s trigger inflammatory responses. If you doubt whether your diet contains many omega-6, stop doubting and be sure that it is. The typical Western diet is oversaturated with omega-6s. Our diet contains 14-25 times more of them than omega-3s. This means a ratio of 14: 1 or 25: 1, which is very far from the ideal 1: 1.

Simple carbohydrates, refined sugars, refined wheat, meat, and dairy products are the most common causes of inflammation. Give preference to brown or black rice, whole grains, buckwheat. Eliminate shelled wheat pasta, white rice, semolina, quick-brew oatmeal, and any other refined grains.

Most Powerful Anti-Inflammatory Foods

Little gradual modifications are typically sustainable, more suitable for the body to adjust to, and may decrease your chances of responding to your old habits. Then instead of emptying your locker, including setting out for the Mediterranean, you can start a small step at a point and begin an anti-inflammatory diet.

By appending anti-inflammatory diets that fight inflammation to your diet, you can start to repair your body outwardly, making any sharp differences by regaining health at the cellular level. When you discover foods that heal your body also satisfy your taste buds, you can eliminate the wrong foods that create inflammation without feeling guilty. Let's get a look at 15 of the best anti-inflammatory foods you can combine with your diet.

1. Green Leafy Vegetables

It is the principal food you require to fill your refrigerator when combating inflammation. Fruits and vegetables are wealthy in antioxidants that restore cellular health as well as anti-inflammatory flavonoids. If you have complexity eating green leafy vegetables, you can make anti-inflammatory vegetable juices to merge greens.

For instance, when you consume biceps, it is abundant in antioxidant vitamins A plus C and vitamin K, which can defend your brain upon oxidative stress induced by free radical damage. Consuming biceps can also shield you from vitamin K deficiency.

2. Bok Choy (Chinese cabbage)

Bok choy, well known as Chinese cabbage, is an excellent source of antioxidant vitamins and minerals. Recent research shows that bok choy also contains more than 70 antioxidant phenolic substances. These include acids called hydroxycinnamic, which are robust antioxidants that remove free radicals. As a versatile vegetable, bok choy can be used in many dishes outside Chinese cuisine, so it is one of the best anti-inflammatory foods.

3. Celery

The benefits of celery in recent pharmacological research include antioxidant and anti-inflammatory properties and preventing heart disease, which helps improve blood pressure and cholesterol levels. Celery seeds (whole seed form, extract form) have impressive health benefits in reducing inflammation and fighting bacterial infections. It is a unique source of antioxidants and vitamins as well as potassium.

Also, balance is the main key to a healthy body without inflammation. An excellent example of inflammation-related mineral balance is celery, the right mix of sodium and potassium-rich foods. Sodium brings liquids and nutrients, while potassium removes toxins. We know that sodium in processed foods is high, but our usual diets are not rich in potassium. Without this pairing, toxins can accumulate in the body and cause inflammation once again. One of the benefits of celery is an excellent source of potassium and antioxidants, and vitamins.

4. Beetroot

The most evident marker of food full of antioxidants is its deep color. The umbrella category of antioxidants contains a large number of substances. In general, they fight to repair cell damage caused by inflammation. The beet gives the signature color of antioxidant betalain and is an excellent anti-inflammatory. Among the benefits of beet when added to the diet, we can see that it increases potassium and magnesium levels that fight cell repair and inflammation.

Beets also contain a small amount of magnesium, and magnesium deficiency is strongly associated with inflammation conditions. While calcium is a vital nutrient, it cannot function well without magnesium in the body. Accumulation of calcium in the body is undesirable. This unpleasant build-up invites, for example, limescale kidney stones, followed by inflammation. However, when a balanced diet is done, calcium-rich anti-inflammatory foods and magnesium allow the body to better process what is consumed.

5. Broccoli

It is no mystery that broccoli is a worthy addition to either diet, the perfect vegetable for healthful eating. It is valuable for the anti-inflammatory diet. Broccoli is excellent in potassium and magnesium, including its antioxidants, which are expressly potent anti-inflammatory factors.

Broccoli holds essential vitamins, flavonoids, and carotenoids and is a significant root of antioxidant power. They go together to decrease oxidative stress inside the body and to inhibit chronic inflammation, including cancer development.

6. Blueberries

Quercetin, which is found in citrus, olive oil, and dark fruits, is a flavonoid (a useful substance or phytonutrient common in fresh foods) that fights inflammation and even cancer. The presence of quercetin is part of the health advantages of blueberries. In a study seeking IBD treatment, noni fruit extract was used to influence intestinal flora and colon damage by inflammatory diseases. Due to the effects of the extract, quercetin produced significant anti-inflammatory effects.

Another study discovers that consuming more blueberries slowed down cognitive decline and improved memory and motor functions. In this study, scientists believed that these results were due to blueberry antioxidants, which prevent the body from oxidative stress and reduce inflammation.

7. Ananas

Generally, when taken as a supplement, quercetin is coupled with bromelain, a digestive enzyme, one of pineapple's benefits. After years of use as part of an anti-inflammatory food protocol, bromelain is observed to have immune modulation capabilities. I.e., it helps to regulate the immune response that generates unwanted and unnecessary inflammation.

Pineapple also helps to improve heart health because it contains an active bromelain enzyme. Pineapple is nature's answer to those who struggle with blood clotting and take an aspirin a day for those who want to reduce the risk of a heart attack. Bromelain has been found to stop blood platelets from sticking together or accumulating on blood vessels' walls (known causes of heart attacks or strokes).

The benefits of pineapple, high in addition to other disease-specific antioxidants that help prevent the formation of vitamin C, vitamin B1, potassium, including manganese supply. Pineapple is full of phytonutrients (plant nutrients), which are useful in addition to many medicines to reduce the signs of some of the most common diseases we see today.

8. Salmon Fish

Salmon is an outstanding source of indispensable fatty acids, and it is estimated one of the most fabulous omega-3 foods. The omega-3 is the joint active anti-inflammatory agent that demonstrates consistently decreasing inflammation, including reducing the requirement for anti-inflammatory drugs.

The analysis explains that omega-3 fatty acids decrease inflammation and reduce the risk of persistent diseases like heart disease, skin cancer, and arthritis. Omega-3 fatty acids remain concentrated inside the brain and are necessary for cognitive and behavioral function.

Between anti-inflammatory foods, fish and meat are essential components. One of the risks of farm fish is that they do not include the same nutrients as naturally fed fish.

9. Bone Water

Bone juices contain minerals in forms that your body can easily absorb; calcium, magnesium, phosphorus, silicon, sulfur, and others. These include chondroitin sulfates and glucosamine. It is used as additional substances to reduce inflammation, arthritis, and joint pain.

When patients suffer from leaking bowel syndrome, they are advised to consume many bone glasses of water containing collagen and amino acid proline and glycine, which may help improve the damaged cell walls of the leaking intestine and the inflammatory bowel.

10. Walnut

When you follow a diet that does not have much meat, nuts, and seeds meet your protein and omega-3 needs. To get anti-inflammatory nutrients, you can add omega-3 rich walnuts to green leafy salads with plenty of olive oil or eat a handful of walnuts between meals.

Phytonutrients help prevent metabolic syndrome, cardiovascular problems, and type 2 diabetes. Some plant nutrients in walnuts are not found in other foods.

11. Coconut Oil

Much can be written about how herbs and oils work together to form anti-inflammatory partnerships. Lipids (oils) and spices are strong anti-inflammatory compounds, especially coconut oil and turmeric components. A study in India found that antioxidants in coconut oil reduce high inflammation levels and improve arthritis more quickly than medical drugs.

Also, oxidative stress including free radicals is the two main causes of osteoporosis. Coconut oil is a leading natural cure for osteoporosis because its benefits include combating such free radicals with high antioxidants levels.

The use of coconut oil, you can easily use in the kitchen as well as topical preparations. As heat-resistant oil, it is an excellent choice for sauteed anti-inflammatory vegetables.

12. Chia Seed

Fatty acids found in nature are more balanced in our typical diets than those we usually consume. For example, Chia seeds contain omega-3 and omega-6, which should be consumed with each other.

Chia contains essential fatty acids alpha-linolenic and linoleic acid, mucin, strontium, minerals containing vitamins A, B, E, and D, antioxidants containing sulfur, iron, iodine, magnesium, manganese, niacin, and thiamine.

Chia is a seed that can reverse inflammation, regulate cholesterol, and lower blood pressure, which is incredibly beneficial for heart health. Also, by reversing oxidative stress, one is less likely to develop atherosclerosis while regularly consuming chia seeds.

13. Flax Seed

Flaxseed, an excellent source of omega-3 and phytonutrients, is full of antioxidants. Lignans are unique fiber-related polyphenols that provide antioxidant benefits for anti-aging, hormone balance, and cellular health. Polyphenols enhance the growth of probiotics in the intestine and help eliminate yeast and Candida Fungus in the body.

Before using flaxseed with your anti-inflammatory foods, grind it in a mill to ensure that your digestive system can easily access the seeds' benefits.

14. Turmeric

The prime component of turmeric is curcumin, an active anti-inflammatory ingredient. Turmeric, documented its impacts against inflammation in several cases, has been confirmed to be invaluable in anti-inflammatory nutrition.

While curcumin is among the significant anti-inflammatory and anti-proliferative agents within the world, aspirin (Bayer, etc.) and ibuprofen (Advil, Motrin, etc.) have been discovered to have no sound effects.

Because of its noble anti-inflammatory qualities, turmeric is extremely useful in assisting people in treating rheumatoid arthritis (RA). A study from Japan assessed its correlation with interleukin (IL), an inflammatory cytokine connected in the RA process. It found that lead "significantly decreased these markers of inflammation.

15. Ginger

Used in fresh, dried, or extracts, ginger is another immune modulator that helps reduce inflammation caused by overactive immune responses.

Ayurvedic medicine has revealed that ginger can improve the immune system before the recorded date. Ginger is believed to be effective in increasing your body temperature, helping to disperse toxin accumulation in your organs. Our body is good at cleaning the lymphatic system, which is the sewer system.

Ginger's health benefits include reducing inflammation in allergic and asthma diseases.

Inflammatory Foods to Avoid

When you diet with anti-inflammatory foods, you naturally begin to eliminate pro-inflammatory foods and substances. There is nothing as satisfying as a diet rich in whole foods.

The primary suspects are saturated and Trans fatty acids. These fats in processed foods increase inflammation and risk factors for obesity, diabetes, and heart disease.

Omega-6 oils that exceed the balance of omega-3 create inflammation in the body. Unfortunately, the University of Maryland Medical Center says, "A typical diet contains 14-25 times more omega-6 fatty acids than omega-3 fatty acids.

Simple, refined sugars and carbohydrates are more culprits than foods that cause inflammation. Limiting refined foods is an essential factor in an anti-inflammatory diet. All grains can replace refined carbohydrates because whole grains are essential food sources. By using fermented yeasts, you can break down nutrients and gain better access to the body.

Also, establishing a regular physical activity routine can help prevent the occurrence or recurrence of systemic inflammation. An active life activated by anti-inflammatory foods and is not limited to processed toxic compounds can free you from inflammation.

Chronic inflammation shortens life expectancy, accelerates aging, and promotes degenerative diseases. This menu will help you to lower it.

Explaining the inflammation is simple: remember the redness, heat, and swelling that accompany a good blow or injury. That is acute inflammation. It responds to aggression in medical terms, be it an infection, a wound, or a toxic substance. Our immune system sets it in motion to slow the progression of damage and, in a second phase, restore tissue and eliminate waste. This process is extinguished in days or months and is usually more or less localized.

But there is also chronic inflammation, which we do not realize, and that is the major of diseases like cancer, diabetes, and cardiovascular diseases, among others. When the inflammation persists overtime beyond what is necessary and stops responding to the therapeutic purpose, it becomes destructive.

This chronic inflammation is a much more complicated process that ends up becoming a dysfunction and works the way for the appearance of chronic diseases such as diabetes, osteoporosis, cardiovascular diseases, fibromyalgia, or cancer. It becomes a silent threat, as it is not obvious as the acute one. Its symptoms are misleading and diffuse and can affect several tissues at once.

4 Weekly Plan For Your Anti-Inflammatory Diet

The secrets of fighting inflammation are to exercise, not stress, sleep well, be in touch with nature and follow an anti-inflammatory diet.

In this menu that we propose below, foods rich in substances that reduce inflammation and promote cell repair abound. To enhance the effect of any of these recipes, add green tea, ginger, and turmeric to your menu at your discretion.

MONDAY

• Breakfast: fasting, apple juice, celery, cucumber, and beet. After half an hour, pure hot cocoa a cup with almond milk and coconut sugar. Add strawberries or bundled cherries.

• Food: as a starter, spinach and lettuce salad with alfalfa or leek sprouts, carrots, pumpkin, and avocado seeds, seasoned with olive oil and fermented soy sauce. As the main course, a lentil stews with chard, peppers, and tomatoes.

- Dinner: a vegan tortilla with chickpea flour, spinach, garlic, and turmeric.

TUESDAY

- Breakfast: fasting, apple juice, carrot, lemon, and celery. After half an hour, a papaya and apple smoothie along with a slice of homemade bread with flax and olive, avocado, or sesame oil.

- Food: as a starter, beet and tomato gazpacho with garlic and sesame oil. As the main course, steamed broccoli and squash, seasoned with a dressing of herbal salt, turmeric, pepper, sunflower seeds, and olive oil.

- Dinner: a vegetable hamburger on sauerkraut, carrot, and curry.

WEDNESDAY

- Breakfast: fasting, a juice of cucumber, orange, and celery with spinach and many mints. After half an hour, and oatmeal muesli with sesame seeds, raspberries, chia, Brazil nuts, and hazelnuts.

- Food: as a starter, a zucchini cream with leeks, coconut milk, and sesame seeds. As the main course, a quinoa salad with pomegranate, cucumber, and beet, seasoned with marinated garlic oil, dried tomatoes, and saffron.

- Dinner: some tofu tacos with chopped almonds and turmeric.

THURSDAY

• Breakfast: fasting, apple juice, pomegranate, and lemon. After half an hour, a slice of homemade almond bread, with psyllium and poppy seeds.

• Food: as an entree, an avocado and pineapple cake with a bite of Brazil nuts, salt, pepper, olive oil, and pumpkin seeds. As the main course, an amaranth soup with fried onion, tomato, pepper, and zucchini, seasoned with ginger and cloves.

• Dinner: good lettuce and spinach with strawberries, nuts, sprouts of leek, and beets. Sprinkle with beer and chia yeast.

FRIDAY

• Breakfast: fasting, a juice of kiwi, spinach, and lettuce. After half an hour, a milkshake of hemp, banana, cinnamon, and cocoa milk accompanied by a buckwheat toast with tahini.

• Food: as a starter, cream of broccoli with onion, bean sprouts, and pumpkin seeds. As the main course, white rice with carrot, dried tomato, garlic, pepper, artichoke, and olive oil.

• Dinner: a plate of tofu with natural tomato sauce, garlic, basil, and black olives.

SATURDAY

Therapeutic fast: based on vegetable broth (onion, leek, thistle, seaweed, and a pinch of seawater) and infusions such as chamomile and green tea spiced to taste and sweetened with stevia.

Optional: light dinner at sunset and breakfast the next day as late as possible (semi-fast).

SUNDAY

A free diet with organic foods and a moderate glycemic index.

What Do Vegans Eat?

A vegan diet plan is free of animal products. The obvious examples are meat, fish, chicken, dairy (animal milk, yogurt, cheese, butter...), eggs, honey, gelatin, and animal broth. "What do you still eat?!" is the most frequently heard spontaneous uplifting question. Well ... seitan stew with fries, vegetable stews, tofu scramble, pancakes, lasagna, risotto, pizza ... From fast food to whole foods, there is something for everyone. The range of vegan cuisine is varied and immense: vegetables, fruit, grains, legumes, nuts, seeds, and herbs. They exist in a huge variety, and you can combine them endlessly in delicious dishes. If you delve into the vegan kitchen, you will find that you have absolutely nothing to lose!

But there's more. Nowadays, many foods from the typical Western diet can be found in a fully vegetable version or can easily be made yourself.

The vegan pantry:

Cereals: there is a huge variety of cereals; think of wheat in the form of bread, pasta, and rice. You can also go on a macrobiotic tour with cooked grains such as millet, barley, and rye.

Legumes: lentils and beans are cheap and an ideal source of protein. With lentils, you make tasty dahl or lentil burger. With beans, you prepare tasty burgers and spreads, and they fit very well in stews and chilies. You can find them very cheaply in the supermarket.

Nuts and seeds: nuts can be a little more expensive, but luckily you never need large quantities of them. Seeds are a lot cheaper. For example, with sunflower seeds, you can make a delicious "cheese sauce." Or you can sprinkle them in your salad, well for some extra proteins.

Seitan, tofu, tempeh: three classic protein sources. Seitan is regularly used to replace meat in classic dishes such as pot roast, marinated on skewers, or as minced meat in a vegan kebab wrap.

Not everyone is immediately won over for the taste of tempeh, although the smoked version can appeal too many.

With tofu, you can go in all directions: marinated fried tofu cubes, as quiche filling, stir tofu, fried tofu fritters... you name it. There are the regular solid tofu and the slightly more liquid "silken" or silk tofu.

Egg substitutes: any pastry can be made without an egg. Possible substitutes are silken tofu, ground linseed or chia seed, apple sauce, egg-replacer, vegetable yogurt, ripe banana... Instead of organizing an egg recipe yourself; you better opt for an existing vegan version. Be sure to try our delicious vegan brownie.

Dairy substitutes: vegetable milk, yogurt, pudding, and cream are for sale in every store. There are varieties based on soy, oats, rice, almonds, hazelnuts, cashews, and so on. Some organic shops and specialty shops have ready-made vegan whipped cream, and you will find Alpro "soy cream to beat" with some luck in the supermarket.

Nowadays, you can find vegan cheese in many supermarkets and organic stores. One is delicious as a slice on a sandwich, the other ideal on a pizza. There are many different types; try as many as possible to discover your favorite. The real kitchen heroes can experiment with making vegan cheese themselves based on cashew nuts and tofu, for example.

Vegan ice cream is also on the rise.

Interesting ingredients:

Noble yeast flakes: the panacea for vegans. It does not only taste like cheese but also provides extra vitamins. Sprinkle them over your spaghetti or process them into parmesan, cheese sauce, pesto... anything you want to give a cheese flavor. Also, read our blog post about noble yeast.

Black salt or Kala counterfeit: thanks to the light sulfur flavor perfect for giving dishes an egg taste. Use it, for example, in tofus cramble, vegan egg lettuce, or even in veganaise.

Soy sauce: provides an extra savory taste. Variants such as tamari, shoyu, or ketjap manis are readily available.

Bouillon: useful for seasoning dishes. Make them yourself, or buy 100% vegetable broth powders and cubes.

Coconut (milk): use it in your favorite curry, to make ice cream, or as whipped cream. You can go many ways with coconut.

Condiments: such as ketchup and mustard, are fortunately usually vegan.

Sweeteners: in vegan desserts, liquid sweeteners such as agave or maple syrup are often used. In Europe, most sugars are almost always vegan.

Cocoa and chocolate: fondant chocolate is not always vegan these days; manufacturers often put milk products in it to reduce costs. To be sure, it is best to check the ingredients list. Certain brands sell vegan milk chocolate and even white chocolate.

Baking powder, baking soda, corn starch, arrowroot: necessary ingredients for baking and/or binding sauces.

Pitfalls

Unfortunately, animal products are often used in food that you would not expect immediately. For example, many vegetarian burgers contain cheese or eggs (Quorn bv.).

In addition, misleading labeling can cause problems. For example, on the packaging of many baking and roasting products, it says "vegetable" or "vegetable product," but they still contain animal fats or milk components. The only reliable indication is the VEGAN logo. For products without a vegan mention, it is advisable to read the ingredients list. It is useful to know that milk whey, milk powder, butterfat, and whey powder are ingredients of animal origin. Cocoa butter and lactic acid are vegan again.

Some additives, listed by name or E-number in the ingredient list, are of animal origin. An example is flour and bread improver L-cysteine (e-920), made from chicken plumes, pig, and sometimes even human hair.

If animal substances were used during the food production process, vegans would also try to avoid them. For example, gelatin and protein are used to clear certain drinks - such as some beers, wines, and fruit juices. On the Barnivore website and with the Vege tipple app, you can look up a lot of drinks to see if they are vegan.

Anti-Inflammatory Diet Day 1 [Vegan]

If you want to reduce inflammation in your body or keep it low, you can try a week filled with anti-inflammatory foods, and meals like these can also be found in my anti-inflammatory diet one day menu. Just like losing weight on a Vegetable Diet menu plan, you can "stretch" the days by making larger portions of the dishes and repeat the day in terms of food.

This day is around 1500 calories, including the 4 snacks and sourdough bread with the soup as indicated on the menu. 1500 calories are sufficient if you want to lose weight, are smaller, and/or less active. The meals provide a large number of anti-inflammatory substances. When you need more calories, you take larger portions; you can eat until you are satisfied instead of paying attention to the precise portions, or you can add some healthy foods such as fruit, whole grains, vegetables, and legumes.

Chia Breakfast Pudding [350 cal.]

Chia pudding is a delicious, quick meal that can be both breakfast and dessert. Chia seeds are a great source of omega 3, a very important element in an anti-inflammatory diet. Healthy fats, antioxidants, and fibers keep us full and satisfied for a long time. I have added a scoop of green powder here; you can also use matcha or cocoa powder. It becomes slightly sweeter with a few drops of stevia or a tablespoon of maple syrup. (approx. 350 calories)

Lunch is an easy blended soup. Blended soups are rich in nutrients; they can be raw or cooked, or what I do most, half and half. I often add some steamed broccoli or peas. This recipe is raw, but you can add steamed vegetables to taste or some white beans for extra protein and filling. The green leafy vegetable is a great source of anti-inflammatory properties and is rich in antioxidants. (Approx. 185 calories) Serve with two slices of whole-grain sourdough or whole-grain crackers topped with a few slices of avocado and slices of tomato.

The evening meal is a bit of an old-fashioned feeling meal, comfort food: a creamy cauliflower parsnip puree, quinoa burger, red cabbage, and apple salad, and lamb's lettuce. The mash is so delicious... it also has a little potato and a tablespoon of tahini through it to make it soft and creamy. (approx. 417 calories)

Red cabbage is rich in anthocyanin, a substance that lowers the level of C-reactive protein, a measure of blood inflammation. A handful of berries and half a cup of shredded red cabbage is sufficient for your daily needs.

I always make more food than I think I need for a meal to make sure we have something left for lunch the next day or for another evening meal. I heat the leftovers, pimp it up with fresh vegetables for a quick meal.

Healthy and sweet for after dinner, Golden Milk made with turmeric and a piece of dark chocolate.

Lists Of Anti-Inflammatory Recipes

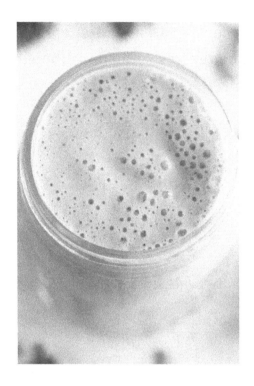

1. Kale smoothie

Kale smoothie, a very satisfying, healthy, and easy to prepare breakfast or drink that is ready in 5 minutes, with only three ingredients.

Servings: 1

Ingredients

- 1 cup of kale (16 g)
- One banana, frozen is better
- 3/4 cup of unsweetened vegetable milk (200 ml), i used almond milk
- One tablespoon of almond butter (optional)
- 1/2 teaspoon ground cinnamon (optional)

- 1 or 2 medjool dates (optional)

<u>Preparation:</u>

1. Pour all the ingredients in a glass mixer and beat until well combined.
2. The smoothie is better freshly made, although you can store it in an airtight container in the fridge for 1 or 2 days.

Nutrition

Serving size: 1calories: 244sugar: 15.2 g

Sodium: 144 mg

Fat: 12 g

Saturated fat: 1.1 g carbohydrates: 34.1 g

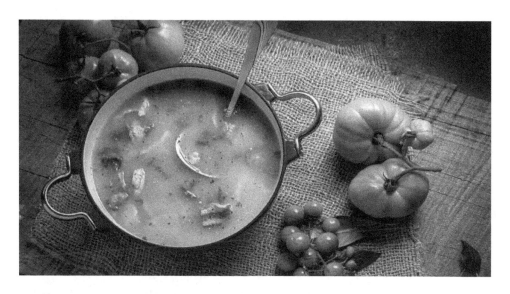

2. Grouper in green sauce

A soft and delicious low-calorie fish easy to prepare and serve in green tomatillo sauce

Yield: 2 servings

Ingredients

- 2 grouper fillets
- Salt and pepper
- 1 tablespoon of olive oil
- For the sauce:
- 2 tomatillos, without the peel
- ¼ cup of pumpkin seeds
- ½ cup of green paprika, without seeds or veins
- ½ cup of coriander leaves only
- ½ of a jalapeño, without seeds or veins
- ½ cup of parsley leaves only
- ½ teaspoon fresh thyme
- 3 garlic cloves

- ¼ cup of fish stock
- 1 pinch of salt

Preparation:

1. In a medium saucepan with water at the time, add the tomatillos and boil 1 minute. Stir and place in the blender.
2. In a medium skillet, add the seeds and toast on low, medium heat for 1 to 2 minutes or until golden brown. Remove and place in the blender.
3. Pour the rest of the ingredients. Blend well.
4. Pour out the sauce into the pan and then cook over medium heat for 1 minute.
5. Dry the fish fillets with the paper towel and salt and pepper to taste.
6. In another wide pan, add the olive oil and let it heat over medium-high heat.
7. Place the steaks and let them brown, 3 to 4 minutes on each side. Serve with the sauce.

Nutritional Information:

340 Cal

24% 19g Carbs

40% 14g Fat

36% 28g Protein

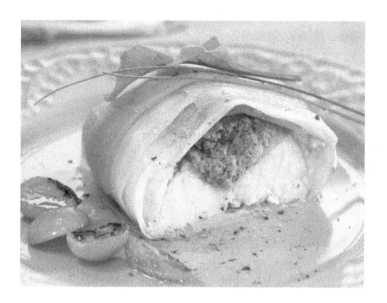

3. Monkfish and spinach parcels

Time preparation: 45 minutes

The sea fish provides plenty of iodine and protein. Both ensure a smooth flow of metabolism. The spicy-tasting leek is very rich in zinc and thus has a wound-healing an immune-boosting effect.

Ingredients

For four portions

- 1.7 oz. spinach
- salt
- 2 bars leek
- Two big carrots (300 g)
- 21.1 oz. monkfish
- One organic lemon
- 10.5 oz. seelachsfilet
- 3.5 oz. of soy cream
- 1.7 oz. cottage cheese (0.3% fat)

- Pepper
- 6.1 inch fish stock (glass)
- 8.8 oz. yellow or red cherry tomatoes
- 1 tbsp. olive oil
- Four red sorrel orchard leaves at will
- ¼ bunch chives

Preparation

1. Clean, wash and drizzle the spinach in boiling salted water and let it collapse in 1-2 minutes. Remove spinach, chill cold, squeeze well, chop and chill.
2. Clean the leeks cut in length and wash. Separate the leaves from each other and add to the boiling salted water for 2 minutes. Then remove cold quench and dab dry.
3. Clean and peel the carrots, cut lengthways into thin strips and add to the boiling salted water for 3 minutes until soft. Remove, chill off cold and dab carrot strips dry.
4. Wash monkfish fillet and pat dry. Lay the bottom of an ovenproof mold slightly overlapping with the leek and carrot strips. Place the monkfish filet in the middle of it.
5. Rinse the lemon hot, rub dry, rub the skin and squeeze juice. Cut the salmon filet into small pieces and puree with soy cream, cottage cheese and spinach to a fine mass. Season the mixture with salt, pepper, lemon peel, and juice, spread on the fillet and beat the vegetable strips over the fish from both sides.
6. Add seelachsfilet, fish stock and cook the monkfish fillet in a preheated oven at 180°C (160°C convection, gas: stage 2-3) for about 30 minutes.

7. In the meantime wash and halve cherry tomatoes. In a frying pan, add olive oil fry the tomatoes in it for about 5 minutes over medium heat.
8. Wash red sorrel orchard leaves and chives and shake dry. Cut monkfish fillet in leek and carrot clove into four pieces and arrange with tomatoes, lettuce leaves, and chives.

Nutritional Information:

Calories: 351 kcal

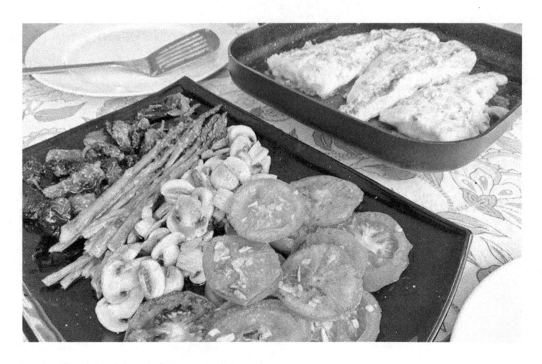

4. Grilled Hake and Vegetables Recipe

This recipe for fresh hake fillets and grilled vegetables is a good combination and a good option for a healthy meal.

Preparation: 10 mins

Cooking Time: 15 mins

Number of Serving: 2

Ingredients for four people:

- 4 fresh hake fillets
- 1 bunch fresh asparagus
- 5 tomatoes
- 10.5 oz. mushrooms
- 7.05 oz. of standard peppers
- 4 crushed garlic cloves

- 1.4 oz., of pure virgin olive oil Arbequina
- Salt to taste
- 1 lemon

How to make the recipe for grilled hake and vegetables

1. Start the oven at 150 ° C
2. Split the lemon in two and with a half sprinkles the hake. Reserve
3. Clean tomatoes, asparagus, mushrooms and standard peppers with water, dry with paper towels.
4. Slice the mushrooms and sprinkle with the other half of the lemon, set aside.
5. Cut the tomatoes into slices a centimeter thick, set aside.
6. Cut the hard part of the asparagus, reserve.
7. Put the roasting pan on the fire, when it has been heated, sprinkle with olive oil and put the asparagus, leave a few minutes, turn around, leave a few more minutes, take out and put on a suitable baking sheet.
8. On the same plate, roast the mushrooms a few minutes on each side, remove and put on the tray with the asparagus.
9. In the same plate place the tomato slices, spread over half the crushed garlic and salt to taste, let it roast for a few minutes and turn it over, let it do a few more minutes, remove and place on the tray with asparagus and mushrooms. Insert the tray into the oven to keep it warm,
10. On the same plate (put a little more oil if necessary) Roast the fresh hake fillets, add salt to taste, leave about five minutes on each side, remove and leave on another tray or plate inside the oven.
11. In a skillet sprinkled with oil, brown the other half of crushed garlic and heat it over the hake fillets.

12. In the same pan that the garlic has browned, add the standard peppers, add salt on top and leave a few minutes turning them occasionally. Remove and place in the vegetable tray.
13. Serve right away.

Nutritional Information:

Calories 92

Fat 1.77g

Carbs 0.17g

Protein 17.79g

5. Asparagus and green pea's salad

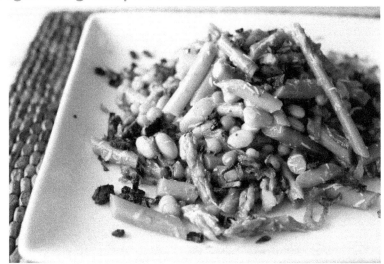

Ingredients

- 1/2 of bunch (8 ounces) asparagus
- 1 1/2 cups of shelled English peas, blanched
- 1/4 cup of fresh mint leaves (you can tear it, if large)
- 1/4 cup of chopped toasted almonds, plus more for serving
- Two tablespoons extra-virgin olive oil
- Two tablespoons of rice-wine vinegar
- Kosher salt and freshly ground pepper

Preparation

1. Trim asparagus. Thinly slice on a strong bias. Toss with peas, mint, almonds, oil, and vinegar. Season with salt and then add pepper, and serve, topped with more mint and almonds.

Nutritional Information:

Calories   87.5

Total Fat	4.1 g
Saturated Fat	1.8 g
Polyunsaturated Fat	0.3 g
Monounsaturated Fat	1.7 g
Cholesterol	9.2 mg
Sodium	685.8 mg
Potassium	212.1 mg
Total Carbohydrate	8.1 g
Dietary Fiber	1.8 g
Sugars	2.2 g
Protein	5.1 g

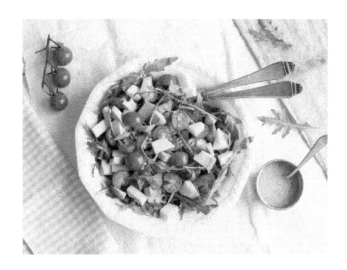

6. Rocket salad with mango, avocado and cherry tomatoes

Time preparation: 15 minutes

Although avocados contain a lot of fat, because in addition to plenty of vitamin E score the green fruits with healthy polyunsaturated fatty acids, Mango has its yellow color due to the plant pigment beta carotene, which is a precursor of vitamin A, which is vital for healthy eyes. The cell-protecting lycopene from tomatoes completes the essential substance package.

<u>Ingredients</u>

For four portions

- 1 tbsp. lime juice
- 2 tbsps. white balsamic vinegar
- 2 tbsps. rapeseed oil
- 2 tbsps. olive oil
- 1 tsp. honey
- 1 tsp. medium hot mustard
- Salt

- Pepper
- Three handful rocket (120 g)
- 200 g cherry tomatoes
- One ripe mango
- Two avocados

Preparation

1. For the vinaigrette, whip lime juice with balsamic vinegar, rapeseed and olive oils. Whisk in honey and mustard and then season with salt and pepper.
2. Wash the rocket and spin dry. Wash tomatoes and halve. Peel the mango, slice the pulp from the core and dice it. Halve the avocados, core them, remove the pulp from the skin and dice them as well. Add cherry tomatoes, ripe mango, avocados - all the salad ingredients inside a bowl with the vinaigrette and spread on four plates.

Nutritional Fact

Calories: 306 kcal

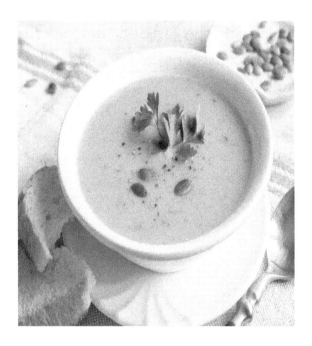

7. Pumpkin cream

Ingredients:

- 1 pumpkin
- 2 onions
- 2 cloves of garlic
- 1 tablespoon butter
- Laminated almonds to decorate

Serves: 1 Person

Preparation:

1. Cut the squash into pieces and salt and pepper.
2. Bake the pumpkin at 180º C until it is soft.
3. Caramelize onions over low heat with the butter.
4. Fry the previously chopped garlic.

5. Blend the pumpkin with the garlic and onion. Add little water if needed, so that the consistency of cream remains.
6. Garnish with rolled almonds.

Nutritional Value

Calories: 49

Carbs: 12 grams

Fiber: 3 grams

Protein: 2 grams

Potassium: 16% of the RDI

Copper, manganese and riboflavin: 11% of the RDI

Vitamin E: 10% of the RDI

Iron: 8% of the RDI

Folate: 6% of the RDI

Niacin, pantothenic acid, vitamin B6 and thiamin: 5%

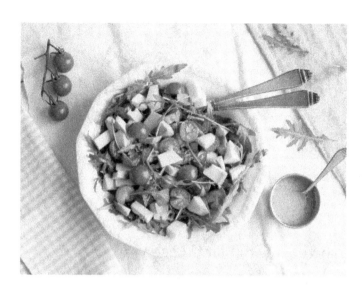

8. Rocket salad with mango, avocado and cherry tomatoes

Time preparation: 15 minutes

Although avocados contain a lot of fat, because in addition to plenty of vitamin E score the green fruits with healthy polyunsaturated fatty acids, Mango has its yellow color due to the plant pigment beta carotene, which is a precursor of vitamin A, which is vital for healthy eyes. The cell-protecting lycopene from tomatoes completes the essential substance package.

Ingredients

For four portions

- 1 tbsp. lime juice
- 2 tbsps. white balsamic vinegar
- 2 tbsps. rapeseed oil
- 2 tbsps. olive oil
- 1 tsp. honey
- 1 tsp. medium hot mustard

- Salt
- Pepper
- Three handful rocket (120 g)
- 200 g cherry tomatoes
- One ripe mango
- Two avocados

Preparation

1. For the vinaigrette, whip lime juice with balsamic vinegar, rapeseed and olive oils. Whisk in honey and mustard and then season with salt and pepper.
2. Wash the rocket and spin dry. Wash tomatoes and halve. Peel the mango, slice the pulp from the core and dice it. Halve the avocados, core them, remove the pulp from the skin and dice them as well. Add cherry tomatoes, ripe mango, avocados - all the salad ingredients inside a bowl with the vinaigrette and spread on four plates.

Nutritional Fact

Calories: 306 kcal

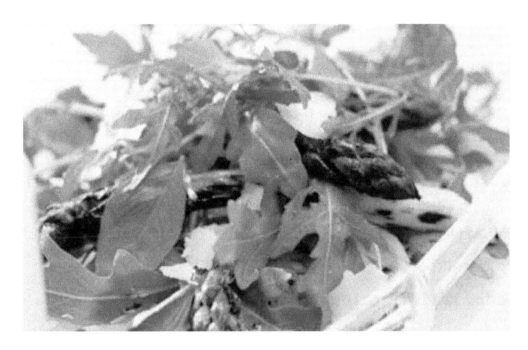

3. Grilled asparagus salad with parmesan

4 people

Preparation time: 15 min.

Cooking time: 6 min.

Ingredients

24 asparagus

- Basting oil
- 75 g arugula leaves.
- 1 bunch fresh basil, chopped
- 3 tablespoon (s) of olive oil
- 2 tablespoon (s) balsamic vinegar
- Salt and freshly ground black pepper
- 175 g parmesan cheese, shaved

Preparation

1. To prepare a grilled asparagus salad with parmesan:

2. Peel the asparagus from the tip to the base and remove the hard part of the stem.

3. Brush them with the oil and grill them on the barbecue grill directly, at medium speed, for 5 to 6 minutes. Turn them over once halfway through cooking and let cook until the marbling due to the grill. Let cool and cut into pieces.

4. Mix the salad leaves, the chopped basil and the asparagus in a salad bowl.

5. Separately prepare a small vinaigrette by mixing olive oil, balsamic vinegar, salt and pepper.

6. Just before serving it, season the salad with the vinaigrette and sprinkle with Parmesan shavings.

7. Here is grilled asparagus salad with parmesan

8. Also enjoy our slimming recipes!

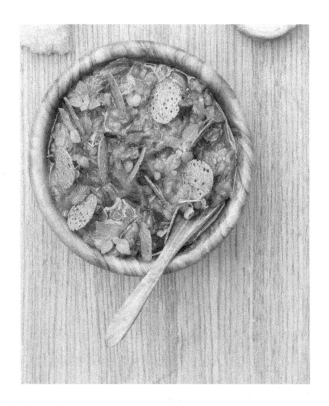

4. Vegan chakchouka

It's even better by roasting a few peppers to give the recipe a little smoky side.

2 people

Preparation time: 40 mins.

Cooking time: 130 mins.

Ingredients

- 3 yellow peppers
- 3 red peppers
- 3 green peppers

- 5 tomatoes
- 2 sweet onions
- 1 bouquet of garni (thyme and bay leaf)
- 1 clove of garlic, peeled
- Espelette pepper.smoked paprika
- Flat parsley
- Fresh coriander
- Olive oil
- Salt, freshly ground pepper

Preparation

1. Bake the peppers inside the oven at 200 ° C / th. 6-7 for 10 minutes, then peel them, scoop them out and cut the flesh into thin strips.

2. Peel the tomatoes and then slice them into large dice. Slice the onions.

3. Pour 10 cl of olive oil into a casserole dish. Brown the onions. Then add the Espelette pepper pepper strips, the bouquet garni, the crushed garlic clove, salt, pepper, a hint of and smoked paprika. Simmer for 2 hours before adding the diced tomatoes, parsley and chopped cilantro.

4. Serve the chakchouka with toast.

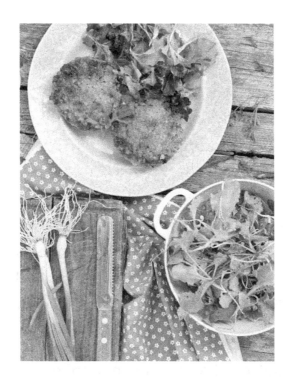

5. Vegetable croquettes

6 people

Preparation time: 30 MIN.

Cooking time: 25 MIN.

Calories: 171 CAL / PERS.

Ingredients

- 1 zucchini
- 2 apples earth
- 1 broccoli
- 150 g fresh peas
- 1 vegetable bouilloncube

- 1 egg (optional)
- 2 tablespoons (s) tablespoons flour of peas Chick
- 5 sprigs of fresh parsley
- 1 tablespoon (s) of olive oil
- 1/2 teaspoon cumin powder
- Salt and pepper

Preparation

1. Peel the potatoes. Detail the broccoli in florets. Coarsely cut the zucchini. Cook all the vegetables in a large volume of water with the bouillon-cube. 20 minutes for potatoes, 10 minutes for broccoli, 8 minutes for zucchini and peas.

2. Pass these vegetables through the potato masher. Finely chop the parsley.

3. In a bowl, beat those egg with the chickpea flour, cumin and parsley. Add salt and pepper. Add the mashed vegetables.

4. Form small vegetable croquettes between your hands.

5. Brown them for 5 minutes in a very hot pan with the olive oil.

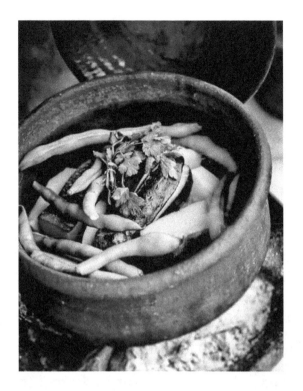

6. Tagine of vegetables with spices

4 People

Preparation Time: 20 Min

Cooking Time: 35 Mins

Calories: 351 Cal / Person

Ingredients

- 2 onions
- 2 tomatoes
- Olive oil
- 1 eggplant
- 200 g snap

- 4 apples earth with firm flesh
- 3 turnips
- 4 carrots
- 1/4 pumpkin
- 1 teaspoon (s) of turmeric and ginger
- 1 teaspoon (s) and 1/2 of paprika and cinnamon
- 1/4 bunch of parsley and coriander

Preparation

1. Peel, seed and slice the tomatoes into small dice.

2. Peel and chop the onions. In a casserole dish, brown them with 3 tsp. olive oil and spices.

3. Taper the snow peas. Cut the eggplant in 4. Peel the other vegetables, cut the carrots into sticks, turnips and potatoes in 2 and the pumpkin into pieces. Put everything in the casserole dish with the herbs; add water, salt and pepper. Cover and simmer 30 minutes.

THE TRICK

Serve with steamed semolina.

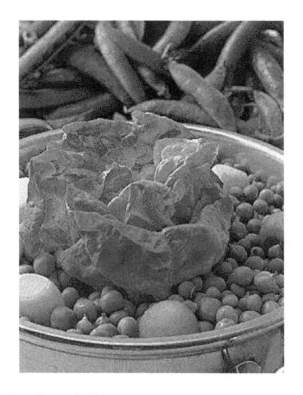

7. Little Peas, the French Way

4 People

Preparation Time: 20 Min.

Cooking Time: 30 Min.

Ingredients

- 1 kg of peas
- 6 onions
- 1 heart of lettuce
- 2 sugar cubes (optional)
- 60 g butter or 2 carrots (optional).bouquet garni
- Salt pepper

Preparation

1. Shell the peas when putting them on the fire or keep them cool in the air.

2. In a thick-bottomed saucepan, place the lettuce heart, peas, onions, sugar, spices and bouquet. Pour 2 cm of cold water, cover, put on medium heat. As soon as boiling is reached, hold it for 15 minutes. Add the butter; simmer over low heat until cooked.

3. If you have just picked peas from your garden, cook them directly in the butter over low heat.

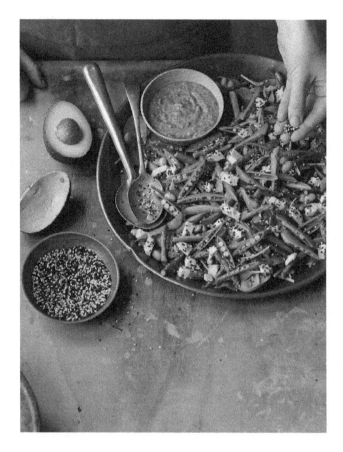

8. Gourmet pea, edamame, and green asparagus salad

4 People

Preparation Time: 25 Min.

Cooking Time: 2 Mins.

Ingredients

- 1 bunch of green asparagus
- 1 tablespoon (s) of olive oil
- 400 g gourmet peas
- 300 g edamame (Japanese beans)
- 300 g baby spinach

1/2 avocado

The sauce

- 1/2 avocado
- 4 tablespoon (s) of coconut milk
- 1/2 teaspoon (s) of honey
- 1/2 green chili
- 1/2 bunch of basil
- 1/2 bunch of coriander
- 3 tablespoon (s) soy sauce
- 4 tablespoon rice vinegar

Preparation

1. Rinse and cut the tips of 1 bunch of green asparagus. Trim the tails into 1 cm sections.

2. Brown everything for 2 minutes in a pan with 1 tsp. olive oil.

3. In a bowl, cover 400 g of gourmet peas and 300 g of edamame (Japanese beans) with boiling water.

4. Mix well the flesh of 1/2 avocado, 4 tsp. coconut milk, 1/2 tsp. honey, 1/2 green pepper, leaves of 1/2 bunch of basil and 1/2 bunch of coriander, 3 tsp. soy sauce and 4 tsp. rice vinegar.

5. In a large dish, mix 300 g of spinach leaves, rinsed and wrung out, the beans and the drained peas, as well as the hash browns. Add the flesh of 1/2 avocado cut into small pieces and the avocado sauce. Decorate with basil and coriander leaves.

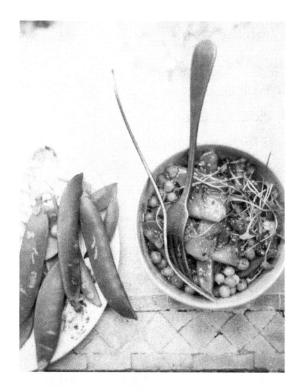

9. Pea salad, gourmet peas, grapefruit

A fresh, crunchy and fruity starter.

6 People

Preparation Time: 20 Min

Cooking Time: 10 Min

Calories: 1 Cal / Pers.

Ingredients

- 1 pink grapefruit
- 800 g shelled peas
- 200 g gourmet peas

- 2 fresh onions with the stem
- 1 tray of sprouted seeds
- 1 drizzles of olive oil
- 1 dash of apple cider vinegar
- 1 tablespoon old-fashioned mustard
- Seeds sesame toasted

PREPARATION

1. Peel the grapefruit and collect the flesh (without the white skin), as well as the juice.

2. Steam peas 3-4 minutes and gourmet peas a little more.

3. Mix the mustard in a salad bowl with the grapefruit juice, olive oil, vinegar, salt and pepper. Add the chopped onions with the stem, the vegetables and the grapefruit flesh. Mix well, sprinkle with sesame and sprinkle with sprouted seeds.

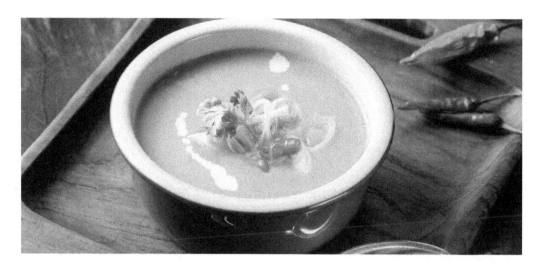

10.Thai Pumpkin Soup

Creamy pumpkin soup with a hint of Thailand: coconut milk, ginger, and chili.

Ingredients

- 0.10 oz. Coconut Oil
- 17.6 oz. Pumpkin
- 14.1 oz. Carrots
- 1piece Spring Onion (50 G)
- 1piece Small Chili
- 1piece Clove Of Garlic
- 0.19 oz. Ginger (30 G)
- 1TL Turmeric
- 19.6 Inches Vegetable Stock
- 15.7 inches Coconut Milk
- 5leaves Thai Basil
- 1piece Lime Leaf
- Prize Salt
- EL Soy Sauce

- Heap Spoon Of Coconut Oil
- Prize Black Pepper
- 1EL Lime Juice
- Fresh coriander to serve

Preparation

1. Cut off the pumpkin drink. Peel pumpkin as needed hollow out the pumpkin and weigh it. Use the same amount of carrots. Peel carrots. Cut pumpkin and carrots into large pieces. Peel ginger and turmeric. Finely chop the spring onion, chili, ginger, turmeric, and garlic.
2. Heat coconut oil in a saucepan. Fry spring onion, ginger, chili, turmeric, and garlic. Add carrots and pumpkin and roast without browning. Add soup and coconut milk, add basil and lime leaf. Bring to a boil, add basil and lime leaf. Simmer on a flame for about 15 minutes until the vegetables are tender. Prick vegetables with a needle. If the vegetables slip off easily, it is soft.
3. Remove lime leaf and basil. Puree the soup with a hand blender.
4. Season it with a little salt, add pepper, soy sauce, and lime juice. Serve with a little coriander.

Nutrition Information

Total Carbohydrate: 29.5 g

Dietary Fiber: 2.9 g

Sugars: 5.6 g

Protein: 5.4 g

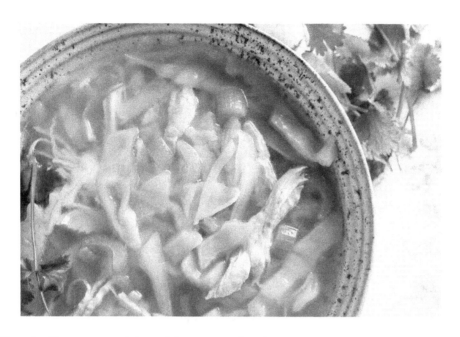

11. Dry belly soup with cabbage and celery

The ingredients have the function of detoxifying the body, eliminating excess swelling and retention of liquid. Celery is diuretic, the onion has the function of detoxifying, the cabbage has low calories and improves bowel function, and the bell peppers bring satiety and more fiber to the body.

Ingredients:

- 1/2 chopped cabbage
- 6 large chopped onions
- 6 tomatoes chopped without seeds
- 3 stalks of celery
- 2 green peppers
- Salt to taste
- Pepper to taste
- Oregano to taste

Preparation:

1. Wash vegetables and chop as instructed above. Bring all of these ingredients into a pan with water to cover.
2. Let it cook over medium-high heat with the pan semi-capped.
3. Season with salt, pepper and oregano and other spices and herbs you prefer.
4. Cook until the vegetables are tender. Serve immediately.

Nutrition Information

Calories: 165.2

Sugars: 4.1 g

Dietary Fiber: 12.0 g

Total Fat: 1.8 g

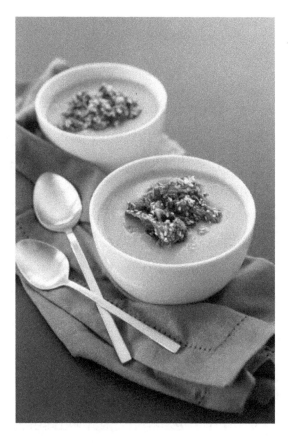

12. Dry Soup Recipe for Pumpkin Belly

Being a source of fiber, the pumpkin helps to cause a feeling of satiety avoiding excessive consumption. Also, the pumpkin is low calorie: 100 grams contains only 40 calories. Make use of this ingredient to lose weight. Ginger helps to speed up metabolism by being thermogenic.

Ingredients:

- 1/2 Japanese Pumpkin
- 0.19 inch ginger, without chopped peel
- 1 chopped onion
- 3 cloves garlic, crushed
- 3 stalks of holy grass
- 1 1/2 l of water

- Olive oil to taste

Preparation

1. Wash the pumpkin in running water. In a pan, put 2 cups water, the pumpkin and lightly cook over medium heat for 10 minutes.
2. Meanwhile, wash, peel and slice the ginger. Peel garlic and onion cut the onion into 4 parts.
3. Transfer pre-cooked squash to a board and, with the vegetable peeler, remove the peel. Reserve the cooking water. Cut the pumpkin into cubes and return to the pan with the water. Add the ginger, the garlic, the onion, the holy grass and the rest of the water. Bring to the medium heat and cook with the pan covered for 40 minutes.
4. After this time, remove the stalks of holy grass. Transfer to the blender and beat everything. Season with little salt and pepper to taste return the soup to the pan to heat and serve them.

Nutrition Information

Total Carbohydrate 16.1 g

Dietary Fiber 4.6 g

Sugars 5.9 g

Protein 7.2 g

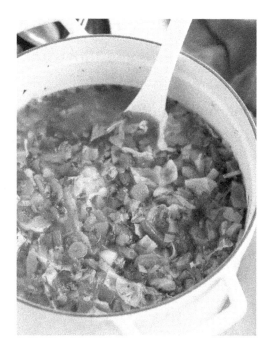

13. Dry belly soup recipe with cabbage

Carrots and cabbage are detoxifying foods and help to deflate. When used in this soup with other low-calorie vegetables, they can promote healthy weight loss.

Ingredients:

- 1 chopped carrot
- 1 chopped turnip greens
- 2 tomatoes chopped without seeds
- 1/2 chopped cabbage into strips
    - oz. of the pod
- 2 cabbage leaves chopped into strips
- 1 chopped onion
- 1 tablespoon of olive oil
- Salt to taste

Preparation:

1. Put the olive oil to heat in a pan. Saute the onion and garlic in a pan. When golden, place the carrot and turnip and cover with 500 ml of water and cook for 20 minutes.
2. Add the remaining ingredients, add more water if necessary and bring to the boil for 10 minutes. Set seasonings and serve!

Nutrition Information

Calories: 57.5

Sugars: 1.8 g

Dietary Fiber: 3.7 g

Protein: 2.5 g

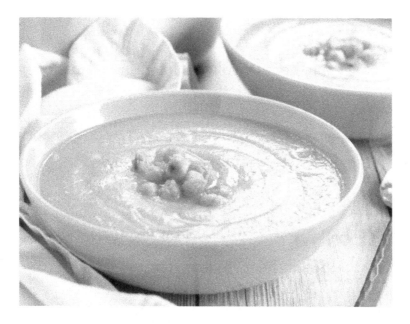

14.   Dry belly soup recipe with sweet potato

Sweet potato is a source of good complex carbohydrates that help you lose weight. By having a low glycemic index, the glucose contained in the sweet potato is released gradually in the body being used as energy and increasing the sensation of satiety.

Ingredients:

- 1 tablespoon of olive oil;
- 2 cloves garlic, minced;
- 1 medium chopped onion;
- 3 tomatoes skinless and chopped seeds;
- 2 chopped zucchini;
- 1 medium sweet potato chopped;
- 2 cups chopped spinach
- Chopped parsley to taste
- 1 liter of water
- Salt to taste

Preparation:

1.   Inside a saucepan, heat the olive oil and then sauté the garlic, onion, and tomato.

2.   Add zucchini, peeled and chopped sweet potatoes and spinach and cook for 5 minutes. Add water, salt and cook until tender.

3.   Wait for the soup to simmer and beat in the blender until you get a creamy soup.

4.   Return to the pot to heat, season seasoning if necessary and serve with fresh parsley.

Nutrition Information

Dietary Fiber: 2.6 g

Protein: 3.2 g

Calories: 132.5

Total Fat: 5.3 g

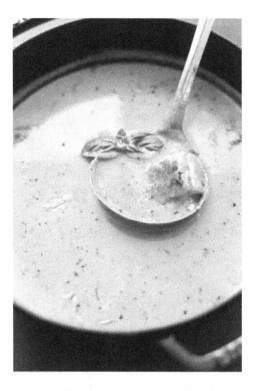

15. Pumpkin Soup

In addition to having just 144 calories and rendering four servings, this recipe for weight-loss soup brings the pumpkin, which is rich in fiber, thus providing a sense of satiety to the body.

Ingredients:

- 2 chuchus
- 1 medium slice of tomato
- ½ small onions
- 2 garlic cloves
- ½ plates (table) of Swiss chard
- 1 stalk of celery
- 1 tablespoon chopped parsley
- 4 small pieces of pumpkin
- 2 ½ cups of water

- 1 teaspoon light salt
- Pepper to taste
- 1 plate (table) of endive
- 2 egg whites

Preparation:

1. Peel and chop all ingredients, except eggs.

2. Put the ingredients in a saucepan, except the endive. Add water, salt, and pepper.

3. Cook until soft, turn off the heat and beat in the blender until a homogeneous mixture is obtained.

4. Add in a saucepan the broth, finely chopped endive strips and whipped whites. Cook a little more, turn off the heat and serve.

Nutritional Information

Protein: 10.1 g

Calories: 164.8

Sodium: 1,060.4 mg

Total Carbohydrate: 22.7 g

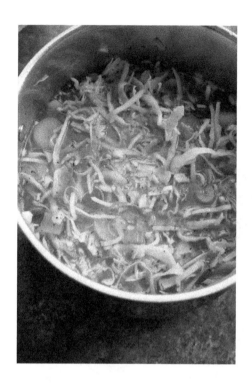

16. Cabbage soup

Replacing dinner with a cabbage soup, which usually has only 71 calories in the size of a cup can help greatly reduce the number of calories in the meal. Also, the ingredient has antioxidants and helps in the digestive process.

Ingredients:

- 2 green peppers
- 6 large green onions
- 15.8 oz. diced tomatoes
- 2 medium carrots
- 1 handful of chopped celery
- 1 packet of onion soup
- ½ chopped cabbage
- 2 cubes of chicken broth
- 2 garlic cloves

- 2 tablespoons chopped parsley
- Salt and pepper to taste

Preparation:

1. To put in a pan the sliced green onion, the cleaned, chopped pepper, the chopped cabbage, the chopped, sliced tomatoes, the chopped carrots, the sliced celery, the garlic, the chopped parsley, the packet of onion soup, the chicken broth and a quantity of water that covers the ingredients.
2. Simmer for two hours. Afterward, turn off the heat and add salt and pepper to taste.

Nutritional Information

71 calories

Sugars: 4.1 g

Dietary Fiber: 12.0 g

Total Fat: 1.8 g

Two Sides Of Inflammation

Inflammation is a carefully engineered healing mechanism for the body. Without inflammation, it is impossible to heal wounds or cure diseases. Even the muscles you worked so hard on could not get bigger and stronger if there were no inflammations. According to the current trend, they could be eliminated by pharmaceutical intervention. The inflammation initiates swelling, allowing proteins, along with white blood cells and antibodies, to enter the damaged area. The same swelling not only allows this antimicrobial defense to be activated but also facilitates the work of growth factors to repair blood vessels and tissues.

So before tackling inflammation, you must first learn to distinguish between the two types of inflammation, since one is generally beneficial, and the other is mostly harmful.

1. Acute inflammations: a beneficial type

Acute inflammation does occur after an injury, such as a cut, bruise, or surgery. They are short-term, localized, and often lead to rapid healing. Acute inflammation is also a major factor in muscle growth. After training, growth factors are supplied to the damaged muscle fibers to accelerate regeneration. Protein molecules - cytokines - first trigger beneficial inflammation and then decrease myostatin levels. The protein myostatin tells the body to stop muscle growth and switch to catabolism, so suppressing myostatin production promotes muscle growth.

Also, acute inflammations awaken dormant satellite cells, triggering their transformation into full-fledged muscle fiber cells. However, by interfering with or stopping the acute inflammation by taking anti-inflammatory drugs such as aspirin, ibuprofen, or naproxen, and even applying ice to the muscles, the swelling that initiates healing can be removed and thus neutralized the effect of post-workout muscle growth.

2. Chronic inflammation: bad type

Chronic inflammation begins as an overreaction to certain stimuli, which are usually harmless. The overreaction can be specific foods, emotional stress, and unhealthy lifestyles, or certain types of bacteria and viruses. The inflammatory response of this type is similar to firing a cannon at a sparrow. The system overreacts, swelling increases, chemical attacks are repeated over and over. After all, in the absence of a real threat, this army of chemicals may even start attacking the body itself, a condition often characterized as an autoimmune disease.

We usually see chronic inflammation in the form of allergies, gluten sensitivity, or one of the hundreds of mysterious diseases that ruin our lives, drain our savings and require unnecessary medical intervention. Chronic inflammation can trigger muscle growth arrest due to increased levels of myostatin, which blocks hypertrophy. Acute inflammation must be maintained or even intensified from time to time, while chronic inflammation must be suppressed and, if possible, eliminated.

The secret cause of inflammation

Few people understand the far-reaching disease-causing consequences of inflammation. They increase insulin resistance even in slender and lean people and negatively affect bone reconstruction. The consequences can even be expressed in the form of incontinence and aggressive behavior. People with depression are 30% more likely to have rarely diagnosed brain inflammation. Inflammation undoubtedly plays a role in cancer. They also actively contribute to obesity, which is a double whammy, as fat itself promotes inflammation.

Inflammation is the main reason dentists are concerned about gum disease. Bacteria living on the gums can travel to the heart and blood vessels, which can cause inflammation in these organs and lead to a heart attack. Strangely, most inflammation can be traced back to the intestines and zonulin, a strangely named protein that regulates the permeability of the intestinal wall, thereby controlling the passage of macronutrients and other molecules through it.

Bowel leaks

Gluten-free people are preoccupied with zonulin. They say that gluten increases zonulin levels and is the source of all troubles. In the intestines, cracks, and crevices randomly begin to open and close, just like a restless Labrador in the back seat, inadvertently stepping on the remote control, opens and closes the garage door.

These cracks and crevices allow protein molecules and even microscopic pieces of food to enter the bloodstream, where they are identified as enemies, triggering an immune response. Inflammation. The intestinal mucosa in people with Crohn's disease and irritable bowel syndrome (IBS) is thickly covered with these gaps, so many of them that it is called "leaky gut syndrome."

However, leaky gut syndrome, or the varying degrees of leaky gut, is not only seen in people with Crohn's disease or IBS. Perhaps anyone suffering from any type of inflammation, systemic or not, has a digestive tract cracked like a country road in Marrakesh. And it's not necessarily caused by gluten. There are other factors as important as or even more important than gluten, whether intolerance is present.

Five horsemen of inflammation

Anything can increase gut permeability and allow stimulants to attack the immune system; however, there are five main culprits:

1. Dietary factors: Alcohol, gluten (sensitive only), processed foods, fast food, etc.
2. Medications: antibiotics, corticosteroids, antacids.
3. Infections.
4. Stress: Physical stress, lack of sleep, or psychological stress, any cause that triggers the release of stress hormones.
5. Hormonal factors: fluctuations or abnormal levels of thyroid hormones, progesterone, estradiol, or even testosterone. (Apparently, naturally, high testosterone levels are normal, but not one that turns you into a roaring bull.)

Any of these factors affect the state of the digestive system, creating small or defective colonies of digestive bacteria. In the absence of a normal bacterial balance, stress hormones and sex hormones increase the intestinal mucosa's permeability. The increased permeability allows foreign objects to enter the bloodstream, stimulating the immune system and leading to local or systemic inflammation.

Prolonged attacks can destroy the intestinal wall. The microvilli that process food are damaged, disrupting digestion. Damaged microvilli are themselves a pro-inflammatory factor. Also, all this bacterial and chemical mess serves as an invitation for SIBO (Small Intestine Bacterial Overgrowth), fungal infections, anything that can seep through cracks in the intestinal mucosa, wreak havoc and release the chemical dogs of chronic inflammation.

Triple attack

The answer must be a multi-pronged attack. You can end stress by eating well, getting enough sleep, and getting more rest. This will stabilize stress hormones and keep the zonulin and fissures in the intestines under control. Fortifications can be built against inflammation in the intestines by creating, deploying, and feeding an army of beneficial digestive bacteria that can withstand SIBO, crush fungi and freeze the parasitic infections that cause inflammation. Finally, we could use supplements and pharmaceutical foods to attack systemic inflammation.

1 - Lifestyle and nutrition

The most effective lifestyle change is getting rid of abdominal fat, a major inflammation source. Just a few weeks of dieting can cause a dramatic decrease in C-reactive protein (a marker of inflammation). Second, it is easy to regulate sleep duration, curb bad habits, regulate sugar levels through diet and supplements such as cinnamon and cyanidin 3-glucoside, and consuming omega-3 fatty acids.

You can also reduce your intakes of potentially pro-inflammatory foods, such as red meat, processed foods, and omega-6 fatty acids (discovered in most vegetable oils and non-organic, grain-fed meats poultry). Whenever possible, try to reduce the intensity of passions at work and home. However, this can be a heroic effort, such as changing jobs, changing partners, or refining your communication skills.

2 - Bacterial Bastion

There is an old meme about the benefits of yogurt consumption and its probiotic contribution to the digestive bacteria population, but this is not a complete strategy. Eating probiotics is like planting a seed but not giving it sun, water, or nutrients. Bacteria multiply and die. They need to be fed, and this is where we need prebiotics. We all have a different bacterial environment, inhabited by various microorganisms. If you imagine your digestive tract in the form of an African jungle, then your neighbor has the jungle of South America. Both are inhabited by birds, mammals, insects, and snakes, but these are completely different species of the creatures mentioned. But among all these conditional tigers, lions, and bears, there are two desirable in every personal jungle: lactobacilli and bifidobacteria.

Fortunately, regardless of the jungle's specific inhabitants, these two critters eat almost the same food, which we call prebiotics. Most of this food is found in indigestible carbohydrates such as inulin, fructooligosaccharides (FOS), and galactooligosaccharides (GOS). We do not assimilate them, but lactobacilli and bifidobacteria eat them.

Suppose you suffer from inflammation (like most of us). In that case, you should first populate your digestive tract with good bacteria by consuming good old sauerkraut every day, which can be found in the refrigerators of the vegetable department. One serving of kale contains about the same amount of bacteria as you'd hope to get from a whole can of probiotic capsules. Of course, you can consume other foods, such as yogurt and the like, but it is quite difficult to determine which of them contain a probiotic and not a pseudobiotic.

3 - Supplements and medicines are dietary cruise missiles

To live and eat right is not enough. No matter how "good" you are, inflammation is just waiting to attack. After all, stress or poor quality sleep cannot be eliminated, and some amount of poor nutrition is inevitable. Likewise, environmental stressors such as excess sun, air pollution, cellular communications, and maybe even Hulk gamma rays cannot be ruled out.

Even exercise is an inflammatory factor and can exacerbate bad types of inflammation. Supplements should be part of your anti-inflammatory diet and lifestyle. Of course, there are a lot of them. Opinions vary, but most people should take the following drugs:

17. Fish Oil
18. Curcumin

Both have shown potent anti-inflammatory effects in a wide range of diseases, from cardiovascular diseases to skin cancer.

Take fish oil, for example. Suppose you ask 100 cardiologists about cardiovascular diseases. In that case, the only point on which 99 of them will be unanimous is the preventive properties of fish oil associated with its powerful anti-inflammatory effect. In cases where the blood vessels are lined with low-density lipoprotein (a type of cholesterol), an inflammatory reaction occurs, and white blood cells attack the area. These cells invade the arterial walls and eat up foreign cholesterol, but this can damage the arteries, leading to a heart ailment or stroke. This reaction can be prevented by consuming fish oil or other anti-inflammatory drugs. It could save your life.

Fish oil plays a vital role in the fight against depression. It is believed that the majority of patients with depression or anxiety do not get relief from antidepressant medications. Still, after the inclusion of fish oil in the diet, they significantly improve mood. Here are a few supplements or medications that most people should take:

19. Resveratrol
20. Green Tea
21. C3G
22. Statins

Cyanidin 3-glucoside (C3G) has shown potent anti-inflammatory properties. It also regulates blood sugar levels by improving carbohydrate absorption, which provides an anti-inflammatory effect.

Statins have been added to the list for ideological reasons and to improve the well-being of some people. They are usually prescribed to lower cholesterol levels, which can be considered a dubious practice, but they also save lives, perhaps for a completely different reason. As it turned out, they have anti-inflammatory properties, and it is this characteristic that can be a factor in the prevention of heart attack.

The Influence Of Psychosomatic Factors On The Course Of Digestive Diseases

The problem of the influence of psychosomatic factors on the course of digestive diseases is considered.

"The mystery of the relationship between psyche and soma is an inexhaustible source of scientific research, which integrates the knowledge and efforts of specialists in various fields to solve specific medical and social problems."

The correlation of "somatic" and "mental" has always been important in medical practice. The mental state of a person is closely related to the functioning of the digestive tract system. The prevailing idiomatic expressions reflect this close connection: "the stomach makes you feel afraid," "I feel the liver," "bile temper," etc. The general pathology is abstractly represented as a continuum of these two types of diseases located between the poles of mental and somatic disorders. The whole clinically polymorphic set of psychosomatic disorders is a real pathology. Among psychosomatic disorders, many modern authors distinguish psychosomatic reactions and psychosomatic diseases.

The group of psychosomatic diseases, which is now considered classical, was singled out by one of the founders of the psychosomatic direction, an outstanding American psychotherapist and psychoanalyst of Hungarian origin, F. Alexander. F. Alexander, since the 1930s, worked at the University of Chicago, and this group of diseases was subsequently assigned the name "Chicago Seven," or "Holy Seven" - Holy Seven. A century has passed, and the "Chicago Seven" still lives in the vocabulary of doctors and psychoanalysts. According to F. Alexander, this group includes:

1) A Stomach Ulcer And Duodenal Ulcer;

2) Ulcerative Colitis;

3) Neurodermatitis;

4) Bronchial Asthma;

5) Arterial Hypertension;

6) Hyperthyroidism;

7) Rheumatoid Arthritis.

The list of psychosomatic diseases is steadily changing and supplementing. It has replenished: panic and sleep disorders, cancer, myocardial infarction, irritable bowel syndrome, sexual disorders, obesity, anorexia nervosa, bulimia.

By definition of academician A.B. Smulevich, one of the leading world-renowned clinicians in the field of psychiatry and psychosomatics, "psychosomatic disorders are a group of painful conditions arising from the interaction of mental and somatic factors and manifested by somatization of mental disorders, mental disorders that reflect a reaction to a somatic disease, or development somatic pathology under the influence of psychogenic factors."

There are three types of etiological factors of psychosomatic disorders:

1) hereditary-constitutional - personality-typological features with characteristic logical features of authenticity, hypochondria, hysteroid, depression, paranoia, etc.;

2) psycho-emotional, or psychogenic - acute or chronic external influences affecting the mental sphere: massive (catastrophic), situational acute, situational prolonged, prolonged with persistent mental overstrain (exhausting);

3) Organic - premorbid organic pathology: prenatal and postnatal injuries, chronic sluggish infections, hypoxic-hypoxemic conditions (especially in the vertebrobasilar basin). A person is immersed in his illness, and his mental experiences are focused on painful sensations.

Psychosomatic disorders include:

- Diseases with the main psychosomatic component (peptic ulcer of the duodenum, ulcerative colitis, etc.);

- Organ neuroses - somatized mental disorders;

- Misogyny - pathological psychogenic reactions to somatic disease;

- somatogenic - mental disorders that occur with several severe somatic diseases and are considered in unity.

Psychosomatic disorders cause 36–71% of patients who go to doctors for digestive disorders. However, medical assistance to this contingent of patients is often inadequate. Psychosomatic conditions encountered in the gastroenterological clinic are an urgent problem of our time. In diseases of the digestive system, secondary psychopathological manifestations are absent only in 10.3% of patients. Separate, fragmented asthenic disorders are noted in 22.1% of patients and 67.3% - more complex psychopathological conditions.

According to ICD-10, the following subgroups are classified as somatoform disorders:

- Somatized Disorder;

- Undifferentiated Somatoform Disorder;

- Hypochondriacal Disorder;

- Somatoform Vegetative Dysfunction;

- Chronic Somatoform Pain Disorder;

- Other Somatoform Disorders;

- Unspecified Somatoform Disorder.

Gastroenterology is the closest to psychiatry's therapeutic disciplines since the gastrointestinal tract is a vulnerable zone for the emergence of various psychosomatic diseases. It is believed that the type of people with special gastrointestinal lability, in whom a painful experience and any (positive or negative) emotions leave a noticeable imprint on the digestive system's functions, is quite common.

Organ neuroses in gastroenterology, or functional disorders of the digestive system in combination with borderline mental pathology:

- gastrulae - without any connection with food intake, a mandatory connection with emotional factors and fatigue, characterized by imagery and distinct objectivity;

- Psychogenic nausea and vomiting;

- esophagospasm;

- lump in the throat (globus hystericus);

- aerophagy - persistent, paroxysmal, often loud belching with air;

- Psychogenic halitosis - a patient's false sensation of halitosis;

- dysgeusia - a neurogenic taste disorder, manifested by food-independent and organic nature feeling of bitterness in the mouth;

- glossodynia - a violation of the sensitivity of the tongue, manifested by burning, pressure, or tingling in the tongue and surrounding areas;

- Psychogenic diarrhoea - an imperative urge to defecate, arising, as a rule, in the most inappropriate situation, with the development of a state of anxious expectation of a recurrence of these phenomena ("bear disease," "diarrhoea-alarm clock");

- Constipation with a neurogenic component - increased concern for the act of defecation and the appearance of anxiety in case of delay, fixing the attention to the frequency, quantity, and quality of one's bowel movements.

In December 2014, at the conciliation conference in Rome, new criteria were adopted, and in the fall of 2015, they were first published. The Rome IV criteria' official presentation took place on May 22, 2016, at the symposium as part of the 52nd American Gastroenterological Week (San Diego, USA). All the Roman criteria IV materials are published in a large two-volume manual, and the main articles are in the journal Gastroenterology's specialized issue. The Roman Consensus IV experts have made changes based on multiple studies conducted over ten years. Due to the magnitude of the amendments, a large number of nuances, experts emphasized the most significant of them:

- Instead of the term "functional," the term "Cerebro-intestinal interaction disorders" will now correctly be used. Although it is much more difficult to pronounce this phrase, the meaning of the arising disorders' real pathogenesis is embedded in it, and their mechanism is more precisely defined.

- Officially approved the involvement of microbes and certain foods in the etiological factors of cerebrovascular interaction disorders.

- "Hypersensitive reflux" - a new official medical term for impaired cerebrovascular interaction (such as the nature of functional disorders with clinical manifestations of heartburn); also, terms such as "chronic nausea syndrome" and "chronic vomiting syndrome" can now be used in medical practice.

- "Opioid-induced constipation," "opioid-induced hyperalgesia," "cannabinoid vomiting syndrome" - these are new accepted terms, even though their "functionality of origin" causes some doubts. On the other hand, the new names for the violation of cerebrovascular interaction are much more accurate in meaning in drug use cases than the former term "functional disorders."

• "Violation of the central perception of gastrointestinal pain" has replaced the familiar expression "functional abdominal pain."

• The dysfunction of the sphincter of Oddi now excludes organic pathology but still considers malformations and enzymatic disorders based on pathology. Changes have been made to the approaches to therapy.

• The term "discomfort" was excluded from the definition of "irritable bowel syndrome," which did not convey a diagnostically meaningful meaning and often disoriented the patients themselves. Now, this concept refers specifically to pain at the time of defecation.

• "Syndrome of the intersection of functional disorders" - the simultaneous flow of several functional states or the transition from one to another, such a term is officially approved, which will greatly facilitate the "medical language" both between colleagues and in conversation with the patient.

One section of the presented Roman criteria IV is called the "Biopsychosocial Model of Functional Digestive Disorders." It shows that the development of a functional disorder is influenced by genetic factors and the environment, neuropsychiatric disorders, and changes in the gastrointestinal tract's physiology.

Hereditary factors can influence in several ways. Genetically determined low levels of interleukin-10 (IL-10) in some patients with irritable bowel syndrome (IBS) affect the sensitivity of the mucous membrane of the stomach and intestines. Genetic polymorphism of serotonin reuptake enzymes (5-hydroxytryptamine - 5-HT) can change its level or affect drugs that block 5-HT. Genetic polymorphism acts on a specific protein, which, in turn, affects the central nervous system (CNS) and local nervous regulation at the intestinal level and α2-adrenergic receptors affecting motility. Currently, mechanisms of the central nervous system's hereditary effect on functional gastrointestinal disorders (FGCR) are being studied.

Psychosocial factors are not criteria for the diagnosis of FGCR; however, they act on the axis "brain-gut," which determine the patient's behaviour and, ultimately, clinical manifestations. There are four main areas of influence of psychosocial factors:

1. Psychological stress usually exacerbates the manifestations of FFA and less often causes symptoms in previously healthy people.

2. Psychosocial factors change the patient's behaviour, forcing them to seek medical help more often. Although patients with FFA have many complaints and are concerned about their health, their examination results are within the reference values.

3. FGCR has psychosocial consequences. Chronic pathology, prolonged discomfort, and pain reduce the patient's working capacity and quality of life; complicate interpersonal relationships in the family and at work.

4. Psychosocial effects on the disease, emotional distress, and inadequate consciousness lead, based on feedback, to the symptoms' consolidation and intensification. Patients with severe symptoms begin to show painful pessimism, catastrophism, hypervigilance (increased attention to discomfort), anxiety for their condition, pain perception threshold, and self-esteem decrease. In such cases, behavioural intervention is required (behaviourism studies behavioural reactions).

Motility disorders cannot explain the occurrence of several symptoms of FGCR: functional pain in the chest probably associated with the oesophagus, syndromes of epigastric pain, irritable bowel, and functional abdominal pain.

Visceral hypersensitivity (hypersensitivity) can explain the manifestations of FGCR. Such patients have a low pain threshold of sensitivity (visceral hyperalgesia), which is proved when balloon bowel distension is used, or have increased sensitivity (allodynia). Visceral hypersensitivity can gradually increase in patients with FGCR and, in this case, is called sensitization or increased pain sensitivity to repeated stimuli. In this case, repeated inflation of the balloon in the intestine causes a progressive increase in pain. Hypersensitivity and sensitization can result from damage to the receptors of the sensitivity of the intestinal mucosa and muscular-intestinal plexus as a result of inflammation. Another possible reason is the degranulation of mast cells closely associated with intestinal nerves or increased serotonin activity, which may be due to exposure to bacterial flora or pathological infection. An increase in excitability is possible as a result of central sensitization. As a result, the central inhibitory regulation of visceral afferent impulses is violated, which reduces pain under normal conditions.

Immune dysregulation, inflammation, and impaired barrier function can contribute to the onset of symptoms, but only in the past years has it been shown that half of the patients with IBS have increased activity of inflammatory sphincter of Oddi cells and pro-inflammatory cytokines. In connection with studies of post-infectious IBS and functional dyspepsia (PD), interest in the intestinal membrane's permeability in places of tight joints, in the intestinal flora, and impaired immune function, has increased. This is consistent with evidence that a third of patients with IBS or dyspepsia associate the onset of the disease with an acute intestinal infection.

The role of violation of the intestine's bacterial flora in the occurrence of FGCR requires further study. There is evidence that the ratio of IL-10 and IL-12, characteristic of the inflammatory response in patients with IBS, is normalized with the introduction of Bifidobacteria infantis. These findings are supported by a moderate positive effect of probiotics and antibiotics on IBS symptoms. FGCR depends on food, diet, which, in turn, affects the intestinal microflora.

There are bi-directional interactions of the axis "brain - GIT." External influences (appearance, smell) and internal perceptions (emotions, thoughts) affect gastrointestinal sensitivity, motility, secretion, and inflammation through the central nervous system. In turn, viscerotropic effects are perceived by the brain and affect the sensation of pain, mood, and human behaviour. Positron emission tomography, the functional magnetic resonance imaging, and other studying methods established a relationship between bowel stretching and the activity of certain parts of the brain, and the results in patients with IBS differed from those in the control group of healthy people. Currently, patients' treatment with FGCR is often based on the same enteral and central brain receptors. Active substances include 5-HT and its derivatives,

Removing waste products from the body and clearing the blood is the main responsibility of the kidneys. Also, the kidney plays a crucial role in the excretion of excess water, minerals, and chemicals from the body; it also regulates the balance of water and minerals in the body such as sodium, potassium, calcium, phosphorus, and bicarbonate. Patients suffering from chronic kidney disease may have an imbalance in fluid and electrolyte balance. Therefore, even normal intake of water, table salt, or potassium can cause serious problems in fluid and electrolyte balance.

People with chronic kidney disease should change their diet according to the advice of the physician and dietitian to reduce the burden on the impaired kidney and prevent distress in fluid and electrolyte balance. There is no fixed diet for patients with chronic kidney disease. Each patient is given different nutritional recommendations depending on the clinical condition, stage of renal failure, and other medical problems. It is also necessary to change the nutritional recommendations for the same patient at different times.

The aims of dietary therapy for patients with chronic kidney disease are as follows:

- Reduce the toxic effects caused by excess urea in the blood.

- Maintain the ideal nutrition habit and prevent loss of lean body mass.
- Reduce the risk of cardiovascular diseases.

The general principles of diet treatment for chronic kidney patients are as follows:

- Limit protein intake to 0.8 gm/kg per kilogram per day for non-dialysis patients. Patients on dialysis need a greater amount of protein to compensate for the possible loss of proteins during the procedure. (1.0 to 1.2 gm/kg daily according to body weight)

- Taking enough carbohydrates to provide energy.
- Taking normal amounts of oil. Reduction of butter, pure fat, and oil intake.
- Restriction of fluid and water intake in case of swelling (edema).
- Dietary intake of sodium, potassium, and phosphorus limitation.
- Taking adequate amounts of vitamins and trace elements. A high-fiber diet is recommended.

High-Calorie Intake

The details of the selection and modification of the diet for chronic kidney patients are as follows:

1. High-Calorie Intake

In addition to daily activities, the body needs calories to maintain heat, growth, and adequate body weight. Calories are taken with carbohydrates and fats. The daily normal calorie intake of patients suffering from chronic kidney disease according to body weight is 35-40 kcal/kg. If caloric intake is insufficient, the body uses proteins to provide calories. Such distribution of the protein may cause deleterious effects, such as improper nutrition and increased production of waste materials. Therefore, it is very important to provide sufficient calories to CKD patients. It is important to calculate the patient's daily calorie requirement based on the ideal body weight, not the current weight.

Carbohydrates

Carbohydrates are the primary source of calories required for the body. Carbohydrates, wheat, cereals, rice, potatoes, fruits and vegetables, sugar, honey, cookies, pastry, confectionery, and beverages. Diabetes and obesity patients should limit the number of carbohydrates. It is best to make use of complex carbohydrates that can be obtained from whole grains such as whole wheat or raw rice that can provide fiber. They should constitute a large part of the number of carbohydrates in the diet. The proportion of all other sugar-containing substances should not exceed 20% of the total carbohydrate intake, particularly in diabetic patients. As long as chocolate, hazelnut, or banana desserts are consumed in a limited amount, non-diabetic patients may be replaced with calories, fruit, pies, pastry, cookies, and protein.

Oils

Unsaturated or "good" oils such as olive oil, peanut oil, canola oil, safflower oil, sunflower oil, fish or snack, saturated and saturated fat such as red meat, poultry, whole milk, butter, pure oil, cheese, coconut and animal fat. It is much better than "bad" oils. Chronic kidney patients should limit the intake of saturated fat and cholesterol that may cause heart disease. In the case of unsaturated fat, it is necessary to pay attention to the proportion of monounsaturated fat and polyunsaturated fat. Excessive uptake of omega-6 polyunsaturated fatty acids (CFAs) and a relatively high omega-6 / omega-3 ratio are detrimental, while the low omega-6 / omega-3 ratio has beneficial effects. The use of vegetable oils instead of uniform oils will achieve this goal. Trans fat-containing substances such as potato chips, sweet buns, instant cookies, and pastries are extremely dangerous and should be avoided.

Restriction of Protein Intake

2. Restriction of Protein Intake

Protein is essential for the restoration and maintenance of body tissues. It also helps to heal wounds and fight infection. In patients with chronic renal failure who do not undergo dialysis, protein limitation is recommended to reduce the rate of decrease in renal function and postpone the need for dialysis and renal transplantation. (<0.8 gm/kg daily according to body weight). However, excessive protein restriction should also be avoided due to the risk of malnutrition.

Anorexia is a common condition in patients with chronic kidney disease. Strict protein restriction, poor diet, weight loss, fatigue, and loss of body resistance as well as loss of appetite; this increases the risk of death. High protein proteins such as animal protein (meat, poultry, and fish), eggs, and tofu are preferred. Chronic kidney patients should avoid high protein diets (e.g. the Atkins diet). Similarly, protein supplements or medications such as creatinine used for muscle development should be avoided unless recommended by a physician or dietician. However, as the patient begins dialysis, daily protein intake should be increased by 1.0 to 1.2 gm/kg body weight to recover the proteins lost during the procedure.

Fluid intake

3. Fluid intake

Why should chronic kidney patients take precautions about fluid intake?

The kidneys play an important role in maintaining the correct amount of water in the body by removing excess liquid as urea. In patients with chronic kidney disease, the urea volume usually decreases as the kidney functions deteriorate. Reduction of urea excretion from the body causes fluid retention in the body, resulting in facial swelling, swelling of legs and hands, and high blood pressure.

What are the clues that there is excess water in the body?

Excessive water in the body is called excessive fluid loading. Leg swelling (edema), ascites (fluid accumulation in the abdominal cavity), shortness of breath and weight gain in a short time are indications of excessive fluid overload.

What precautions should chronic kidney patients take to control fluid intake?

To prevent overloading or loss of fluid, the amount of fluid taken on the advice of a physician should be recorded and monitored. The amount of water to be taken for each chronic kidney patient may vary, and this rate is calculated according to the urea excretion and fluid status of each patient.

What is the recommended amount of fluid for patients with chronic kidney disease?

Unlimited edema and water intake can be done in patients who do not have edema and who can throw enough urea from the body. It is a common misconception that, to protect their kidneys, patients with kidney disease should take massive quantities of water and fluids. The recommended amount of fluid depends on the patient's clinical condition and renal function.

Patients with edema who cannot appoint sufficient urea from the body should limit fluid intake. To reduce swelling, fluid intake within 24 hours should be less than the amount of urine produced by the daily body.

In patients with edema, the amount of fluid that should be taken daily should be 500 ml more than the previous day's urine volume to prevent fluid overload or fluid loss. This additional 500 ml of liquid will approximately compensate for the fluids lost by perspiration and exhalation.

Why should chronic kidney patients keep a record of their daily weight?

To track the rise or loss of fluid or to control the amount of fluid in their bodies, patients need to keep a record of their weight regularly. Body weight will remain constant if the instructions for fluid intake are strictly followed. Sudden weight gain indicates excessive fluid overload due to increased fluid intake in the body. Weight gain is a warning that the patient should make more rigorous fluid restriction. Weight loss is usually caused by fluid restriction and the use of diuretics.

Useful Tips for Restricting Fluid Intake

Although it is difficult to limit fluid intake, the following tips will help:

Weigh at the same time every day and adjust fluid intake accordingly.

Calculate accordingly to make a daily intake of the specified amount of fluid. Liquid intake is not only possible with water, tea, coffee, milk, juice, ice cream, cold drinks, soup, as well as watermelon, grapes, cabbage, tomatoes, celery, sauce, gelatin and other foods containing high amounts of water, such as frozen sugary products are also possible.

Note.

Reduce salty, spicy, or fried foods in your diet because these foods can increase your thirst and cause more fluid consumption.

For water only, if you're thirsty. Do not drink as a ritual or drink for everyone's sake. When thirsty, consume only a small amount of water or try ice — sure taking a little ice cube. Ice stays in the mouth longer than water so that it will give a more satisfying result than the same amount of water. Remember to calculate the amount of liquid consumed. To calculate simply, freeze the amount of water allocated for drinking in the ice block.

To prevent dry mouth, gargle with water, but do not swallow the water. Dry mouth can also be reduced by chewing gum, sucking hard candies, lemon slices or mint candies and using a small amount of water to moisturize your mouth.

Always use small cups or glasses to limit fluid intake. Instead of consuming extra water for medication use, take your medicines while drinking water after meals.

The patient should engage himself in a job. Patients who are not engaged in a job often desire to drink water.

Since the person's thirst increases in hot weather, measures to be in cooler environments may be preferred and recommended.

How should the recommended daily amount of liquid be measured and consumed?

Fill the amount of water recommended by the doctor for daily intake into a container.

The patient should keep in mind that he should not take more than the recommended daily intake of fluid.

When the patient consumes a certain amount of liquid except water, the same amount of water should be removed from the container.

It is recommended that the total fluid intake be distributed evenly throughout the day to avoid the need for excess fluid.

This daily repeated method, when applied regularly, contributes to the effective completion of the recommended daily intake and prevention of excessive fluid intake.

Dietary Salt (sodium) Restriction

4. Dietary Salt (sodium) Restriction

Why is low-sodium nutrition recommended for chronic kidney patients?

The amount of sodium in our diet is very important in maintaining the blood volume of the body and controlling blood pressure.

In chronic kidney patients, the kidneys cannot remove excess sodium and fluid from the body, so these two accumulate in the body. Increased amount of sodium in the body causes increased thirst, swelling, shortness of breath, and increased blood pressure.

To prevent or reduce these problems, the intake of sodium in the diets of chronic kidney patients should be restricted.

What is the sodium and salt difference?

Sometimes, the terms sodium and salt are used synonymously. Table salt contains 40 percent of sodium and is sodium chloride. Salt is the primary source of sodium in our diet, but it is not the only source of sodium. There are also different sodium compounds in our foods:

- Sodium alginate: Used in ice cream and chocolate milk.
- Sodium bicarbonate: Used as baking soda or soda.

- Sodium benzoate: Used as a preservative in sauces.
- Sodium citrate: Gelatin is used to intensify the taste of desserts and beverages.
- Sodium nitrate: Used to protect and color processed meat.
- Sodium saccharide: Used as an artificial sweetener.
- Sodium sulfite: It is used to prevent the discoloration of dried fruits.

The compounds above contain sodium and are not salty. Sodium is present in these compounds.

How much salt should be taken?

Typically, the daily salt intake is about 10 to 15 grams (4-6 grams of sodium). Chronic kidney patients should take salt according to the advice of their doctor. Chronic kidney patients with edema (swelling) and high blood pressure are generally recommended to take less than 2 grams of sodium per day.

Potassium Restriction in Nutrition

5. Potassium Restriction in Nutrition

Why is potassium limitation required in the diet of chronic kidney patients?

Potassium is an essential mineral that is necessary for the body to function properly for the muscles and nerves and to keep the heartbeat steady. Normally, the level of potassium in the body is stabilized by consuming potassium-containing foods and excreting excess potassium in the urine. In a patient with chronic kidney disease, excess potassium may not be excreted in the urine sufficiently, which can lead to high levels of potassium accumulation in the blood (known as hyperkalemia). Patients undergoing peritoneal dialysis have a lower risk of hyperkalemia than patients undergoing hemodialysis. The reason for the difference in risk status in the two groups is the continuity of the dialysis process in peritoneal dialysis and the intermittent hemodialysis.

High levels of potassium can cause severe muscle weakness or irregular heart rhythm, which can be dangerous. When potassium is too high, the heart may stop suddenly, and sudden death may occur. A high potassium level can be life-threatening without any noticeable signs or symptoms (hence known as a silent killer).

Conclusion

To avoid problems, we must consume as many unprocessed foods as possible. The best alternative is to switch to a Mediterranean diet that provides a solid dose of omega-3 fatty acids (which can be obtained from sea fish, olives, and nuts).

The menu should not be deficient in herbs and spices: ginger, rosemary, curry, oregano, cayenne pepper, cloves, and nutmeg.

The consumption of vegetables and fruits should be increased. It is especially beneficial to eat spinach, collard greens, broccoli, Brussels sprouts, carrots, beets, onions, and seaweed, rich in anti-inflammatory compounds. Among fruits, dark-colored berries, such as blueberries or blackberries, provide the most.

There should be no shortage of whole grains on the menu. You should eat buckwheat and barley, quinoa, wild and brown rice. If you need to have lunch or dinner with pasta, you should choose made with rye or whole grain flour and cooked al dente. They have a low glycemic index, which is very important for anti-inflammatory nutrition.

Also, experts urge to eat fiber-rich legumes (beans, peas, lentils) and soy products such as tofu. Asian mushrooms, such as shiitake or maitake, will also be helpful to support the immune system.

What to drink to cope with inflammation? First of all, water, but it is also worth drinking tea, especially white and green.

CPSIA information can be obtained
at www.ICGtesting.com
Printed in the USA
BVHW061823230221
600896BV00012B/1622